Evaluation and Management of Autonomic Disorders

Juan Idiaquez • Eduardo Benarroch
Martin Nogues
Editors

Evaluation
and Management
of Autonomic Disorders

A Case-Based Practical Guide

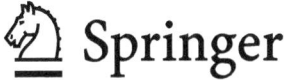 Springer

Editors
Juan Idiaquez
Universidad de Valparaiso
Viña del Mar
Chile

Eduardo Benarroch
Mayo Clinic
Rochester, MN
USA

Martin Nogues
Clinica Fleni
Buenos Aires
Argentina

ISBN 978-3-319-72250-4   ISBN 978-3-319-72251-1   (eBook)
https://doi.org/10.1007/978-3-319-72251-1

Library of Congress Control Number: 2018932421

Printed on acid-free paper

This Springer imprint is published by Springer Nature
The registered company is Springer International Publishing AG
The registered company address is: Gewerbestrasse 11, 6330 Cham, Switzerland

Preface

This book is primarily aimed to general practitioners in the field of neurology, internal medicine, family medicine, and cardiology. Unlike other books on autonomic disorders, this book seeks to provide a brief practical and ready-to-use resort for physicians faced with patients' autonomic complaints.

Using a clinical presentation-based scenario approach, this book allows a rapid access to information required for the evaluation and management of these complex patients.

This book is divided into two parts. Part A includes four chapters that review the anatomy, physiology, and pharmacology of the autonomic nervous system. It also includes the classification, general evaluation, and principles of the management of autonomic disorders. Part B is dedicated to specific clinical autonomic cases that cover autoimmune conditions, neurodegenerative disorders, common peripheral neuropathies, small fiber neuropathies, orthostatic intolerance syndromes, and disorders with autonomic hyperactivity. Each clinical case includes a differential diagnosis, specific tests for the diagnosis, a description of the relevant aspects of the condition, and precise management for each condition.

This book attempts to provide a practical approach for the recognition and management of common autonomic disorders.

Viña del Mar, Chile	Juan Idiaquez
Rochester, MN	Eduardo Benarroch
Buenos Aires, Argentina	Martin Nogues

Contents

Part I
General Principles

Chapter 1
Anatomy, Physiology, and Pharmacology of the Autonomic Nervous System (ANS)

Juan Idiaquez, Eduardo Benarroch, and Martin Nogues

The ANS is a component of the nervous system that has a major role in the maintenance of homeostasis and adaptive responses to external or internal stressors. It innervates all organs of the body, including the eye, the skin, and the cardiovascular, respiratory, gastrointestinal, and genitourinary systems, and functionally interacts with the endocrine, pain, and motor systems. The ANS consists of three subdivisions: the sympathetic, parasympathetic, and enteric nervous systems. The sympathetic and parasympathetic systems each have a central preganglionic neuron in the brainstem or spinal cord and a peripheral neuron in the autonomic ganglia. The preganglionic neurons receive and integrate two types of infor-

J. Idiaquez (✉)
Universidad de Valparaiso, Viña del Mar, Chile
e-mail: idiaquez@123.cl
E. Benarroch
Mayo Clinic, Rochester, MN, USA
e-mail: benarroch@mayo.edu
M. Nogues
Clinica Fleni, Buenos Aires, Argentina
e-mail: mnogues@fleni.org.ar

© Springer International Publishing AG 2018
J. Idiaquez et al. (eds.), *Evaluation and Management of Autonomic Disorders*,
https://doi.org/10.1007/978-3-319-72251-1_1

3

mation, inputs from primary visceral afferents that trigger autonomic reflexes and descending inputs from central autonomic areas that initiate responses to stress, emotion, and other behavioral states. The enteric nervous system consists of neurons located in ganglia within the walls of the gut that participate in local reflexes (Fig. 1.1).

1.1   Central Autonomic Areas

Several interconnected areas of the cerebral cortex, diencephalon, and brainstem control autonomic function brain.

A. The **insular cortex** is the primary visceral sensory cortex. The posterior dorsal insula receives, via the thalamus, inputs from pathways transmitting visceral as well as pain and thermal information. The anterior insula, via its interactions with other cortical areas and the amygdala, is involved in conscious awareness of the bodily sensations.

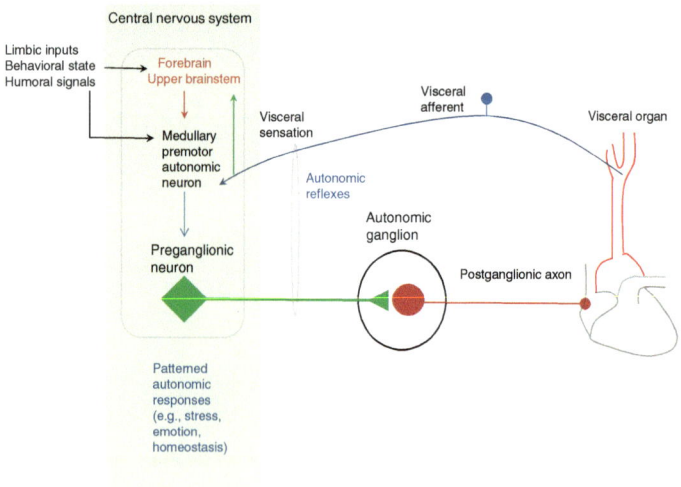

FIGURE 1.1 General organization of the autonomic nervous system

B. The **anterior cingulate cortex** is the cortical autonomic motor area; it includes a rostral portion that is involved in emotional regulation and a dorsal subdivision, which initiates autonomic responses associated with cognitive control, including motivation and decision-making.

C. The **amygdala** is a nuclear complex that has a critical role in emotion and social behavior. It consists of a basolateral complex that integrates information from multiple sensory modalities and is critical for acquisition and consolidation of conditioned responses (including fear) and a central nucleus that initiates autonomic, endocrine, and motor responses to emotion via its inputs to the hypothalamus and brainstem.

D. The **hypothalamus** has a critical role in the generation of integrated autonomic, endocrine, and behavioral responses for maintenance of homeostasis and adaptation to internal or external stimuli. It consists of a periventricular zone that contains nuclei that control hormone secretion by the hypophysis; a lateral zone containing nuclei involved in thermoregulation, osmoregulation, and regulation of feeding, energy metabolism, and reproduction; and a lateral zone that participates in motivated behavior and regulation of the sleep-wake cycle. The main hypothalamic areas controlling autonomic function are the paraventricular nucleus, which is involved in responses to stress, and the lateral hypothalamic area, which is involved in behavioral arousal.

E. **The periaqueductal gray matter (PAG)**, located in the midbrain, integrates descending inputs from the cerebral cortex, amygdala, and hypothalamus with ascending inputs from pathways conveying pain and visceral sensation. The PAG consists of several regions that coordinate motor and cardiovascular responses to stress, are critical for central modulation of pain, and mediate the cortical control of micturition and other visceral functions.

F. The **parabrachial nucleus,** located in the dorsal pons, is a critical integration center that receives visceral, nociceptive, and thermic inputs from the spinal cord and nucleus of the solitary tract and relays this information to the hypothalamus, amygdala, and thalamus. This nucleus also has an important role in control of respiration.

G. **The nucleus of the solitary tract (NTS),** located in the posterior medulla, is the first relay station for visceral inputs from cardiovascular, respiratory, and gastrointestinal receptors conveyed by the glossopharyngeal and particularly the vagus nerves. This nucleus has two main functions: (1) initiation of medullary reflexes controlling blood pressure, heart rate, respiration, and gastrointestinal motility and (2) relay of visceral information to the hypothalamus and other brain areas, both directly and via projections to the parabrachial nucleus. The nucleus off the solitary tract is also the primary relay of inputs from taste receptors.

H. The **ventrolateral medulla** contains several groups of neurons that are critical for cardiovascular and respiratory function. They include sympathoexcitatory vasomotor neurons of the **rostral ventrolateral medulla (VLM)** that project to the intermediolateral cell columns and are critical for control of blood pressure, neurons in the ventrolateral portion of the **nucleus ambiguus** that control the heart rate via the vagus nerve, and neurons of the **ventral respiratory group** extending throughout the medulla and controlling the

I. **The medullary raphe** contains different groups **of** neurons that participate in mechanisms of thermoregulation (responses to cold), automatic ventilation, and pain modulation.

1.2   Organization of the Sympathetic and Parasympathetic Systems

Sympathetic Nervous System

The preganglionic sympathetic neurons are located in the **intermediolateral cell column and the T**1 to L2 segment of the spinal cord. They are organized into different functions controlling cardiac, vasomotor, sudomotor, and visceral effectors. These preganglionic sympathetic subunits receive descending inputs from the hypothalamus and brainstem and segmental inputs from the periphery via dorsal root ganglia afferents. The preganglionic sympathetic neurons control visceral function via projections to two types of ganglia, paravertebral and prevertebral. The **paravertebral ganglia** form the sympathetic chain, which is like a string of beads on each side of the vertebral column, and contain the ganglion neurons that innervate the cranial effectors (including the eye and cerebral blood vessels), skin, and thoracic and abdominal, visceral including the heart, lungs, and gastrointestinal tract. The **prevertebral ganglia** lie anterior to the vertebral column, mostly on the abdominal aorta and its major branches, and innervate all visceral and blood vessels of the abdomen and pelvis, including the rectum, bladder, and genital organs. **A** third effector of the sympathetic system is the **adrenal medulla,** which receives inputs from the intermediolateral cell column and releases epinephrine to the general circulation.

Parasympathetic Nervous System

The preganglionic parasympathetic neurons include two groups, cranial and sacral. The **cranial parasympathetic** neurons occupy the general visceral efferent column of the brainstem and provide inputs from that area carried by cranial nerves to local ganglia that innervate effectors in the face, thorax, and abdomen**,** for example, the **Edinger–Westphal nucleus projects**, via the oculomotor (III) cranial nerve to the ciliary ganglion, which innervates the eye, and the superior and inferior **salivatory nucle**i project, via the facial (VII) and glossopharyngeal (IX) nerve to cranial blood vessels and lacrimal and salivary glands. The **dorsal motor nucleus of the vagus** provides the most widespread parasympathetic output and projects to ganglia located in plexus innervating the heart and respiratory system, as well as intrinsic plexus neurons of the enteric nervous system of the esophagus, stomach, small intestine, ascending, and transverse colon. Neurons in the ventrolateral portion of the **nucleus ambiguus** provide the vagal output to the sinus node and control of heart rate. The sacral parasympathetic neurons are located in the **sacral parasympathetic nucleus** at the S2–S4 levels of the sacral cord and provide inputs to the ganglia innervating the descending colon, rectum, gladder, and genital organs.

Specific Functional Circuits

Control of Blood Pressure

The sympathetic innervation of blood vessels of the limbs and abdomen is critical for the maintenance of blood pressure (BP), particularly in standing position. In addition to this short-term sympathetic mechanism, humoral mechanisms such as the vasopressin and renin-angiotensin-aldosterone system are important for long-term maintenance of BP. The main cardiovascular reflex controlling BP is the **arterial baroreflex.** The arterial baroreceptors respond to pulsatile blood pressure, and they are located in the carotid sinus, innervated by the glossopharyngeal nerve, and the aortic arch, innervated by the vagus nerve, and provide inputs to the NTS. In response to the increase in arterial pressure, inputs from baroreceptors activate neurons of the NTS; these neurons send (1) a direct excitatory input to the cardiovagal neurons of the nucleus ambiguus that decrease the heart rate and (2) indirect inhibitory inputs to the vasomotor neurons of the rostral VLM, which results in a decrease in sympathetic vasomotor tone, vasodilatation, and decrease in peripheral resistance. In contrast, a fall of BP reduces baroreceptor input and NTS activation, leading to increase in heart rate and vasomotor tone. Thus, the arterial baroreflex is critical for the continuous maintenance of BP within a narrow range, and its function is critical to avoid orthostatic hypotension or arterial hypertension. For long maintenance of BP, sympathetic activation of the kidney produces local vasoconstriction, increment of tubular reabsorption of sodium, and stimulation of renin secretion. Other reflexes controlling BP are **cardiac reflexes** and the **arterial chemoreflex**. Stimulation of atrial receptors by atrial distension stimulation increases cardiac sympathetic activity, whereas activation of ventricular receptors by chemical stimulation causes bradycardia and vasodilatation; the arterial chemoreceptors are located in the **carotid body** and are stimulated by hypoxia; the arterial chemoreflex includes sympathoexcitation and increases ventilation.

Control of the Heart

The sympathetic control of the heart involves preganglionic neurons at the T1–T6 segments (primarily T3) and is primarily mediated by the stellate ganglion; the right sympathetic innervates the sinoatrial node and produces tachycardia; the left sympathetic innervates the atrioventricular node and ventricles and increases intrinsic cardiac excitability and myocardial contractility and oxygen consumption. The sympathetic output to the heart is critical to increase cardia output, for example, during exercise. Vagal innervation of the heart originates in the ventrolateral portion of the nucleus ambiguus, which controls the automatism of the sinus node primarily via the right vagus, reduces heart rate, and reduces atrioventricular conduction primarily via the left vagus nerve. The vagal control of the heart rate is modulated by respiration; inspiration reduces the vagal output and produces tachycardia; expiration increases vagal output and elicits bradycardia; this is known as **respiratory sinus arrhythmia**. Therefore, respiratory sinus arrhythmia depends exclusively on vagal modulation of the heart rate. The dorsal motor nucleus of the vagus innervates the ventricles and may reduce ventricular excitability.

Thermoregulation

Maintenance of core temperature of human body depends on (1) thermoreceptors in the skin that detect external temperature via transient receptors' potential channels, (2) neurons in the preoptic area of hypothalamus that detect changes in blood temperature and activate heat loss mechanisms, (3) neurons in the dorsomedial nucleus of the hypothalamus and nucleus raphe pallidus that activate heat production, and (4) output mechanisms mediated by the sympathetic and motor systems. The sympathetic innervation of the skin is critical for thermoregulation. Under a range of ambient temperature, maintenance of body temperature depends on skin vasomotor changes; when temperature increases occur, skin vasodilatation and vasoconstriction occur in cold ambient. When skin vasodilatation is not able to control body temperature rise, sweating occurs, and when skin vasoconstriction is not able to avoid low body temperature, shivering happens.

Control of the Bladder

Storage and elimination of urine are controlled by three spinal inputs, (1) preganglionic parasympathetic sacral neurons that stimulate contraction of the bladder detrusor via the pelvic nerve, (2) lumbar sympathetic neurons that inhibit the detrusor and activate the bladder neck (internal sphincter) via the hypogastric nerve, and (3) somatic motor neurons of the Onuf's nucleus that innervate the external urethral sphincter via the pudendum. The activity of these three outputs is coordinated in an opposite fashion during the two reflexes controlling the bladder, the storage (continence) reflex and the micturition reflex; these reflexes act in a switch-like pattern and are triggered by afferent inputs from the hypogastric and pelvic nerves. The **storage reflex** is a spinal reflex triggered by bladder afferent inputs that occur during bladder filling; this results in the activation of sympathetic and Onuf's nucleus neurons, leading to bladder relaxation and contraction of the internal and external sphincter. The **micturition reflex** is supraspinal reflex triggered when bladder fullness reaches a threshold; increase in afferent activity is conveyed via an ascending pathway to the periaqueductal gray, which sends a projection to the **pontine micturition center** (also known as Barrington nucleus or pelvic organ control center). Neurons from the pontine micturition center send a descending projection to the sacral spinal cord; these projections directly activate the sacral preganglionic neurons, triggering contraction of the detrusor, and indirectly (via interneurons) inhibit the Onuf's nucleus producing relaxation of the external sphincter. Thus, the inputs from the pontine micturition center to the sacral cord is critical for coordination of the parasympathetic and somatic output controlling bladder emptying; interruption of this input leads to detrusor-sphincter dyssynergia. The micturition reflex can be transiently inhibited in response to behavioral or social needs. This requires inputs from the medial frontal cortex, basal ganglia, and anterior hypothalamus to the periaqueductal gray.

Sexual and Reproductive Control

The control of sexual function involves limbic circuits of the cerebral cortex and amygdala, hypothalamus, periaqueductal gray, and autonomic system. Penile erection and clitoral engorgement depend on sacral parasympathetic outflow that produce relaxation of erectile tissue and vasodilatation, mediated principally by nitric oxide. Ejaculation depends on lumbar sympathetic innervation that produces contraction of the smooth muscles of the epididymis, vas deferens, seminal vesicles, and prostate gland. In addition to the autonomic system, endocrine outputs such as prolactin, estrogen, and testosterone have a major role in regulating these functions.

Control of Gastrointestinal Function

Motor and secretory functions depend on bidirectional connection of the central nervous system neurons with the enteric nervous system (ENS), a widespread network of sensory neurons, interneurons, and motor neurons located in the myenteric plexus and submucosal plexus within the wall of the gastrointestinal tract. The ENS contains in total about 200–600 million neurons that participate in local reflexes controlling gastrointestinal motility (peristalsis) and secretion throughout the gut. In addition to local reflexes, the ENS is regulated by extrinsic parasympathetic and sympathetic inputs. Parasympathetic inputs from the vagus nerve are critical to control motility of the esophagus and the stomach, where intrinsic ENS reflexes mostly control the motility of the distal intestine. Sympathetic outputs inhibit motility throughout the gastrointestinal tract.

Control of Effectors in the Eye

The autonomic nervous system controls the diameter of the pupil, accommodation of the lens, intraocular pressure, and lacrimal secretion. The sympathetic innervation of all effectors in the eye originates in the superior cervical ganglion. The parasympathetic innervation of the pupil and ciliary muscle originates from the ciliary ganglia that receive preganglionic input from the oculomotor nerve (CN III). The parasympathetic innervation of the ocular blood vessels and lacrimal gland originates in the pterygopalatine ganglion that receives preganglionic inputs via the facial nerve (CN VII). Normal pupil diameter depends on an active balance between parasympathetic influences producing pupil constriction and sympathetic influences producing pupil dilation. Parasympathetic denervation allows non-balanced sympathetic activity resulting in pupillary dilatation (mydriasis), while sympathetic denervation results in pupillary constriction (miosis). The parasympathetic innervation originates in neurons of the Edinger–Westphal nucleus that send preganglionic axons with the oculomotor nerve (CN III) and relay in the ciliary ganglion in the orbit. Postganglionic axons from the ciliary ganglion innervate the pupil constrictor, as well as the ciliary muscle responsible for accommodation of the lens. Sympathetic innervation consist in a three neuron system, the first neuron is located in the hypothalamus, the second preganglionic neuron in the ciliospinal center (spinal level T1 and T2), and the third postganglionic neuron in the superior cervical ganglia that send axons to the dilator muscle. Both the pterygopalatine ganglia (parasympathetic) and the superior cervical ganglia (sympathetic) control ocular blood flow, as well as intraocular pressure, which on aqueous humor formation is controlled by ciliary body blood, ciliary epithelium, and aqueous humor outflow via a trabecular meshwork and episcleral blood vessels.

Autonomic Neurotransmission

Autonomic Ganglia

The primary autonomic neurotransmitter of the preganglionic neurons innervating both the sympathetic and parasympathetic ganglia, as well as the ENS, is **acetylcholine (ACh),** which produces fast excitation of ganglion cells via ganglion-type nicotinic acetylcholine receptors (nAChRs), which are cation channels permeable to sodium and calcium. Autoantibodies against these receptors produce autoimmune autonomic ganglionopathy, characterized by sympathetic, parasympathetic, and ENS failure.

Sympathetic Neurotransmission

The primary neurotransmitter of essentially all sympathetic ganglion neurons, including those innervating the smooth muscle of the blood vessels, eyes, and viscera and the cardiac myocytes, is **noradrenaline (NA).** The adrenal medulla mediates sympathetic effects via release of **adrenaline** to the general circulation. Both catecholamines act via $\alpha1$, $\alpha2$, $\beta1$, $\beta2$, and $\beta3$ adrenoceptors, which are G-protein-coupled receptors located in the target organs. The $\alpha1$ receptors trigger calcium influx and mediate vasoconstriction as well as contraction of the smooth muscle of the pupil (pupil dilator), bladder neck, and vas deferens. The $\alpha2$ receptors are predominantly presynaptic receptors that inhibit neurotransmitter release, including that of NA (autoreceptors). The $\beta1$ receptors are primarily responsible for the sympathetic stimulation of the heart; the β2 receptors mediated relaxation of smooth muscles leading to vasodilation, bronchodilation, and relaxation of the bladder detrusor (also mediated by β3 receptors). In addition to NA, many sympathetic fibers also release cotransmitters such as neuropeptide Y and adenosine triphosphate, which potentiate the effects of NA. Unlike other effectors, the sweat glands are innervated by sympathetic axons that release ACh; these cholinergic sympathetic axons stimulate sweat secretion via muscarinic receptors.

Parasympathetic Neurotransmission

The primary neurotransmitter of most parasympathetic neurons is ACh, which exerts both excitatory and inhibitory effects via different types of muscarinic receptors. Like adrenergic receptors, muscarinic receptors are G-protein-coupled receptors and include two main subtypes in the autonomic system, excitatory M3 type and inhibitory M2. The M3 receptors mediate all the stimulating effects of ACh on smooth muscles and exocrine glands; they are responsible for pupil constriction, accommodation, lacrimation, salivation, increase of gastrointestinal motility and secretion, and micturition. The M2 receptors mediate the inhibitory effects of the vagus nerve on the heart. Many parasympathetic neurons release other neurotransmitters such as vasoactive intestinal polypeptide and nitric oxide (NO) in addition to or instead of ACh. These neurotransmitters, particularly NO, are responsible for the parasympathetic effects producing smooth muscle relaxation, including vasodilation of cranial and pelvic effectors, relaxation of the esophageal sphincter, gastric accommodation, and penile erection (Table 1.1).

Features of Autonomic Neurotransmission

There are several distinguishing features of autonomic neurotransmission. These include (1) cotransmission, which refers to the release of several transmitters including the classical parasympathetic (ACh) and sympathetic

Table 1.1 Sympathetic and parasympathetic effects

Target	Sympathetic			Parasympathetic		
	Effect	NT	Receptor	Effect	NT	Receptor
Pupil	Dilatation	NE	α 1	Constriction	ACh	M3
Heart	Stimulation	NE	β 1	Inhibition	ACh	M2
Vessels	Constriction	NE	α 1	Dilation	NO	
	Dilation	NO				
	Dilation	Epi	β			
Sweat gland	Stimulation	ACh	M3			
Salivary gland	Variable			Stimulation	ACh	M3
Bronchi	Relaxation	Epi	β	Constriction	ACh	M3
Gastrointestinal motility	Inhibition	NE	α 2, β	Stimulation	ACh	M3
				Inhibition	NO	
Gastrointestinal secretion				Stimulation	NO, VIP	
Bladder detrusor	Inhibition	NE	β	Stimulation	ACh	M3
Bladder neck	Contraction	NE	α 1	Relaxation	NO	
Sexual organs	Ejaculation	NE	α 1	Erection	NO	

ACh acetylcholine, *Epi* epinephrine, *NE* norepinephrine, *NO* nitric oxide, *NT* neurotransmitter, *VIP* vasoactive intestinal polypeptide

(NA) and neuropeptides, ATP, or NO; (2) neurotransmitter interactions at both presynaptic or postsynaptic levels, resulting in functional antagonism between the sympathetic and parasympathetic influences acting on a common target cell; and (3) **denervation supersensitivity**, which is the exaggerated response of a denervated effector cell to small doses of a cholinergic or adrenergic agonist (Fig. 1.2).

Autonomic Pharmacology

Drugs affecting adrenergic or cholinergic transmission are used to manage a wide variety of autonomic disorders. In contrast, blockade of NA or ACh may be responsible for the side effects of drugs used to treat other disorders.

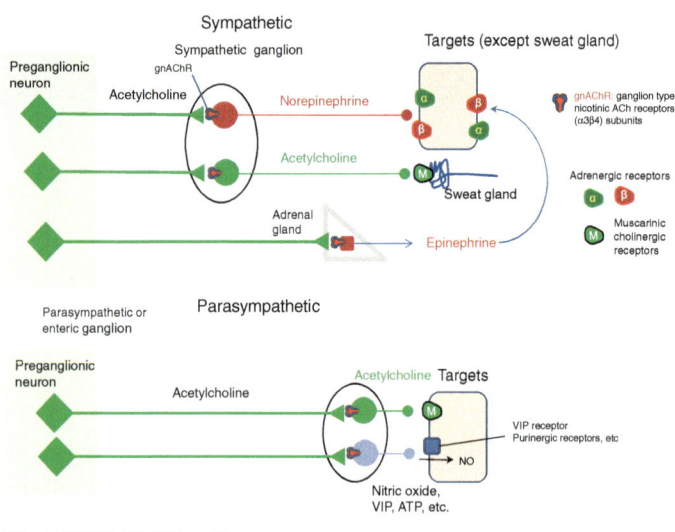

VIP = vasoactive intestinal peptide
ATP = adenosine triphosphate

FIGURE 1.2 Basic autonomic neurotransmission: receptors

Adrenergic Function

Several drugs increase adrenergic transmission via effects on NA synthesis, storage, release, reuptake, and metabolism or via their effects on adrenergic receptors. For example, L-threo-dihydroxyphenylserine (L-threo-DOPS, droxidopa) is a synthetic amino acid converted to NA by L-aromatic amino acid decarboxylase; this drug is used for treatment of orthostatic hypotension (OH). Amphetamine, cocaine, methylphenidate, and atomoxetine inhibit the presynaptic NA transporter responsible for NA reuptake; all these drugs may therefore produce increase in arterial pressure. Midodrine is a prodrug that produces a metabolite that activates α1 receptors and is the first line treatment for OH. Ephedrine and phenylephrine also activate α1 receptors. Clonidine activates α2 receptors and reduces sympathetic activity both at the level of the CNS and presynaptic adrenergic terminals; it is used to prevent episodes of hypertension in the setting of baroreflex failure. Beta-adrenoceptor blockers, such as propranolol, atenolol, metoprolol, and nadolol, are used to treat excessive tachycardia in patients with postural tachycardia syndrome.

Cholinergic Function

Botulinum toxin A blocks proteins that mediate docking of synaptic vesicles and inhibits ACh release; it is used for management of hyperhidrosis, sialorrhea, and excessive bladder activity. In contrast, 3,4-diaminopyridine blocks presynaptic potassium channels and increases ACh release; it improves both muscle weakness and autonomic function in patients with Lambert-Eaton myasthenic syndrome. Pyridostigmine produces a reversible inhibition of acetylcholine esterase and increases synaptic ACh levels at the level of the autonomic ganglia and periphery; it is used as an adjuvant for treatment of OH and gastrointestinal hypomotility. Carbachol, bethanechol, and pilocarpine activate muscarinic M2 receptors. Carbachol is used to treat glaucoma, bethanechol to promote bladder emptying, and pilocarpine to increase lacrimal and salivary secretion. In contrast, drugs such as atropine, oxybutynin, and glycopyrrolate block muscarinic receptors. Atropine is used to treat excessive bradycardia in the setting of cardiac disorder or intoxication with anticholinesterase agents. Oxybutynin is used to treat bladder overactivity and hyperhidrosis; glycopyrrolate is also used to treat hyperhidrosis as well as excessive tracheobronchial secretions.

Adverse Effects of Drugs on Autonomic Function

Many drugs used for treatment of neurologic or psychiatric disorders affect autonomic neurotransmission and produce undesirable side effects. For example, doxazosin and terazosin block off $\alpha 1$ adrenoceptors and are used to relax the smooth muscle of the bladder in patients with obstructive urinary symptoms; however, these drugs may produce OH. Antidepressant such as amitriptyline doxepin, antihistaminic such as diphenhydramine, drugs used to treat movement disorders such as trihexyphenidyl, block muscarinic receptors. In addition to their adverse central nervous system effects, these drugs produce dry mouth, dry eyes, constipation, and urinary retention. In toxic doses, these drugs also produce dilated unreactive pupils, tachycardia, and anhidrosis.

Chapter 2
Classification of Autonomic Disorders

Juan Idiaquez, Eduardo Benarroch, and Martin Nogues

Autonomic nervous system dysfunction may present as hypofunction or hyperfunction and can occur in a wide range of conditions like genetic, neurodegenerative, autoimmune, infectious, metabolic, toxic, and secondary to a nervous system trauma or tumor. The clinical manifestation may be generalized affecting sympathetic, parasympathetic, and enteric systems or localized. Presentation of symptoms may be monophasic, progressive, or episodic. We combined clinical and pathological manifestations in the following syndromes:

J. Idiaquez (✉)
Universidad de Valparaiso, Viña del Mar, Chile
e-mail: idiaquez@123.cl

E. Benarroch
Mayo Clinic, Rochester, MN, USA
e-mail: benarroch@mayo.edu

M. Nogues
Clinica Fleni, Buenos Aires, Argentina
e-mail: mnogues@fleni.org.ar

© Springer International Publishing AG 2018   19
J. Idiaquez et al. (eds.), *Evaluation and Management of Autonomic Disorders*,
https://doi.org/10.1007/978-3-319-72251-1_2

1. Generalized autonomic failure, it can present with a combination of symptoms restricted to ANS dysfunction or autonomic symptoms associated with central and/or peripheral somatic manifestations. Principal causes are listed in Table 2.1. In pure autonomic failure (PAF), a slowly progressive sporadic neurodegenerative disorder, symptoms are restricted to autonomic dysfunction. In multiple system atrophy, progressive autonomic manifestation occurs in combination with parkinsonism, cerebellar ataxia, and/or pyramidal signs. Also in Parkinson's disease, there are motor and autonomic dysfunctions, during the clinical progression of generalized autonomic. Listed in Table 2.2 are causes of generalized autonomic hyperactivity that can present sympathetic or parasympathetic hyperactivity, in Table 2.3 are causes of focal autonomic dysfunction including selective pupillary denervation and restricted sweating dysfunction, and in Table 2.4 are conditions presenting mainly with orthostatic intolerance.

TABLE 2.1 Classification of autonomic failure disorders

Phenotype	Temporal profile	Disorder
Isolated autonomic failure	1. Acute or subacute	Autoimmune autonomic ganglionopathy (AAG)
		Paraneoplastic autonomic neuropathy
	2. Progressive	Pure autonomic failure (PAF)
Autonomic failure associated with parkinsonism, ataxia or dementia	Progressive	Multiple system atrophy (MSA)
		Lewy body disorders: Parkinson's disease
		Dementia with Lewy bodies
Autonomic failure associated with peripheral neuropathy	1. Acute or subacute	Guillain-Barré, porphyria
		Sensory and autonomic neuropathy
		Paraneoplastic neuropathy
	2. Chronic	Metabolic: diabetes mellitus, uremia, vitamin B12 deficiency
		Amyloidosis
		Autoimmune: Sjögren syndrome, systemic lupus erythematosus

		Hereditary
		    Hereditary sensory and autonomic neuropathies (HSAN), familial dysautonomia (HSAN-3)
		    Fabry disease

		Sodium channelopathies
Autonomic failure associated with muscle weakness		Toxic: Alcohol, chemotherapeutic agents
		Infectious: Leprosy, HIV, Chagas disease
		Eaton-Lambert syndrome, myasthenia gravis
		Botulism

TABLE 2.2 Classification of autonomic hyperactivity

Causes	Examples
Diffuses central nervous system	Acute neurologic disorders
Lesion	– Trauma
	– Hypoxia
	– Subarachnoid hemorrhage
	– Brain mass with high IP
	– Acute hydrocephalus
	Autoimmune disorders
	– Limbic encephalitis (VGKC-LGI1)
	– Morvan's syndrome (VGKC-Caspr2)
	– Anti-NMDA receptor encephalitis
	– Stiff man syndrome (GAD or GyR1R)
Focal cortical lesion	Insular stroke
	Temporal lobe seizure
Diencephalic disorders	Fatal familial insomnia
	Episodic hypothermia
Brainstem disorders	Mass lesion
	Brainstem stroke
	Inflammatory lesions
Spinal cord disorders	Autonomic dysreflexia in spinal cord injury
	Inflammatory disorders (NMO)
Peripheral disorders	Guillain-Barré syndrome
	Porphyria
	Baroreflex failure
	Familial dysautonomia

TABLE 2.3 Classification of focal autonomic disorders

System	Clinical manifestation	Disorders
Pupillary lesion		
Sympathetic	Horner (miosis)	Stroke, lung carcinoma, Thyroid tumor
Parasympathetic	Adie (mydriasis)	CN III: stroke, tumor
		Vascular compression
		Peripheral neuropathies
		AAG
Sympathetic sudomotor		
Cardiovagal	Primary hyperhidrosis (palms, soles)	Idiopathic, familial
	Segmental anhidrosis	Spinal cord lesions
		Peripheral neuropathies
		Pure autonomic failure
	Segmental anhidrosis, Adie, areflexia	Ross syndrome
	Hemianhidrosis	Stroke
	Compensatory hyperhidrosis	Spinal cord lesions
		Peripheral neuropathies
		Pure autonomic failure
		Sympathectomy
	Gustatory sweating	Idiopathic
		Secondary:
		Parotid glands lesion
		Peripheral neuropathies
		Parkinson's disease
	Arrhythmias	Epilepsy, stroke
Cranial Secretomotor	Xerostomia Xerophthalmia Crocodile tears	CN VII, palsy
Enteric	Megaviscera	Chagas disease

Table 2.4 Orthostatic intolerance syndromes

Syndromes	Cause
Neurogenic orthostatic hypotension	
Neurally mediated syncope	
1. Vasovagal	Triggers: Postural, emotional distress
2. Reflex syncope	Situational: Micturitional, defecation, other carotid sinus hypersensitivity
Postural tachycardia syndrome (POTS)	Neurogenic POTS
	Hyperadrenergic POTS

Chapter 3
General Evaluation of Autonomic Disorders

Juan Idiaquez, Eduardo Benarroch, and Martin Nogues

The purposes of evaluation of autonomic dysfunction in patients with symptoms and signs suggesting autonomic compromise are the following:

1. Identification of the presence of autonomic symptoms due to autonomic hypo- or hyperactivity (Table 3.1)
2. Assessment of sympathetic and parasympathetic dysfunction with autonomic tests (Table 3.2)
3. Evaluation of patient with general and laboratory test to study specific disorders (Table 3.3)

J. Idiaquez (✉)
Universidad de Valparaiso, Viña del Mar, Chile
e-mail: idiaquez@123.cl

E. Benarroch
Mayo Clinic, Rochester, MN, USA
e-mail: benarroch@mayo.edu

M. Nogues
Clinica Fleni, Buenos Aires, Argentina
e-mail: mnogues@fleni.org.ar

© Springer International Publishing AG 2018
J. Idiaquez et al. (eds.), *Evaluation and Management of Autonomic Disorders*,
https://doi.org/10.1007/978-3-319-72251-1_3

TABLE 3.1 Clinical manifestations of autonomic disorders

System	Autonomic failure	Autonomic hyperactivity
Sympathetic		
Cardiovascular	Neurogenic orthostatic hypotension	Hypertension
		Paroxysmal hypertension
		Tachyarrhythmia
		Takotsubo cardiomyopathy
Sudomotor: focal or generalized	Anhidrosis	Hyperhidrosis
Pupillary	Miosis (Horner syndrome)	Mydriasis
Parasympathetic		
Cardiovascular	Fixed tachycardia	Bradycardia, asystolia
Pupillary	Mydriasis (Adie syndrome)	
Urogenital	Urinary retention	Urinary urgency
	Erectile dysfunction	Incontinence
	Ejaculatory dysfunction	
Cranial secretomotor	Sicca syndrome:	Sialorrhea, lacrimation
	Dry mouth, dry eyes	
Enteric		
	Gastroparesis	Abdominal cramps
	Constipation	Diarrhea, vomiting
	Intestinal pseudo obstruction	

TABLE 3.2 Autonomic function tests

Function	Effector pathway	Neurotransmitter (receptor)	Test
Parasympathetic cardio vagal	Nucleus ambiguous-cardiac ganglion	Acetylcholine (M2)	Heart rate (HR) response to deep breathing Valsalva ratio 30:15 ratio
Sympathetic vasomotor	Rostral ventrolateral medulla-intermediolateral cell column (IML)-sympathetic ganglion	Norepinephrine (α1)	Blood pressure (BP) and HR change during head-up tilt BP response during the Valsalva maneuver BP response to handgrip Cold pressor test
Sympathetic sudomotor	Hypothalamus-IML-sympathetic ganglion	Acetylcholine (M3)	Thermoregulatory sweat test
	Peripheral sympathetic axon to sweat gland		Quantitative sudomotor axon reflex tests
	Peripheral axon to sweat gland		Sympathetic skin response

Table 3.3 General and specific tests

General laboratory tests: plasma glucose, hemoglobin A1C, creatinine, liver function tests, vitamin B12, folate, methylmalonic acid, complete blood count, sedimentation rate, urinalysis

Tests based on specific syndromes	Acute or subacute autonomic failure (AF)	AF associated with parkinsonism, ataxia, or dementia	AF associated with peripheral neuropathy
	Nerve conduction EMG	MRI (putamen and/or pontocerebellar atrophy)	EMG and nerve conduction studies
	Autoantibodies: Ganglionic Ach R Paraneoplastic SSA SSB	Polysomnography: REM behavior disorder Stridor, central apnea	Autoantibodies: Ganglionic acetylcholine receptor, paraneoplastic SSA SSB
		Urodynamics: Post-voiding residua Supine and standing catecholamines	Protein electrophoresis and immunofixation including light chains in plasm and urine Skin biopsy Salivary gland biopsy Abdominal fat aspirate

| Special tests in specific circumstances | Suspect underlying malignancy: CT chest, abdominal, pelvis Testicular ultrasound PET scan | Psychometric testing SPECT or PET scan FMRP for fragile X syndrome Cardiac MIBG Fragile X syndrome | Suspect underlying malignancy: CT chest, abdominal, pelvis Testicular ultrasound PET scan |

Chapter 4
Principles of Management of Autonomic Disorders

Juan Idiaquez, Eduardo Benarroch, and Martin Nogues

Main considerations are: (1) Patient education that must consider a detailed explanation about each common and atypical autonomic symptom, including a basic report of the causative mechanism, the factor that can precipitate or aggravate the manifestations. (2) Discontinuation of potentially causative drugs. (3) Non-pharmacological approach includes diet guiding, daily activities program and physical methods. (4) Pharmacological therapy: pathophysiological based drug management is required. In Table 4.1 is listed non-pharmacological management of OH, drug treatment of OH is listed in Table 4.2. Non-pharmacological and pharmacological treatment for gastrointestinal manifestation is listed in Table 4.3 and for genitourinary dysfunction is listed in Table 4.4.

_____
J. Idiaquez (✉)
Universidad de Valparaiso, Viña del Mar, Chile
e-mail: idiaquez@123.cl

E. Benarroch
Mayo Clinic, Rochester, MN, USA
e-mail: benarroch@mayo.edu

M. Nogues
Clinica Fleni, Buenos Aires, Argentina
e-mail: mnogues@fleni.org.ar

© Springer International Publishing AG 2018
J. Idiaquez et al. (eds.), *Evaluation and Management of Autonomic Disorders*,
https://doi.org/10.1007/978-3-319-72251-1_4

31

Table 4.1 Non pharmacological therapy for OH

Approach	Main considerations	Additional points
1. Patient education	Learn about OH symptoms:	Symptoms reflect hypoperfusion of tissues
	Light headedness, visual neck pain, Presyncope, syncope	Symptoms may present different degree of severity patients with asymptomatic OH may present subtle symptoms due to aggravating factors on standing in the morning, after meals to check post prandial hypotension, at night to checksupine hypertension
	Cognitive slowing, fatigue	
	Leg pain and weakness, walking	
	Orthostatic dyspnea or angina	
	Daily control of blood pressure	
	Aggravating factors of OH	Measures to adopt: to get up slow from bed urinate in sitting position
	Postural hypotension	

Valsalva maneuver	Avoid when it is possible:
Hot environment, exertion	Cardiovascular drugs:
Prolonged recumbence	Nitrates, Calcium channel blockers, Beta blockers,
Drugs may low blood pressure	Diuretics, ACE inhibitors
Mainly in elderly subjects	Antiparkisonian drugs:
	Levodopa, combined therapy
	Psychotropic drugs:
	Benzodiazepines, Serotoninergic and
	Tricyclic antidepressant, Chlorpromazine
	Clozapine, Risperidone
	Anesthetic drugs:
	Lidocaine, Propofol, Halothane

(continued)

Table 4.1 (continued)

Approach	Main considerations	Additional points
2. Diet	Adequate hydration	2–2.5 L of water per day
		Rapid ingestion of 500 mL of tap water
	Sodium intake	Up to 10 g of salt daily
		Check 24 h urinary sodium concentrations
	Type and frequency of meals	Carbohydrates rich meals provoke splanchnic
		Vasodilatation, small quantity of meals every 4 h
		Eat carbohydrates at night. Avoid alcoholic drinks
3. Physical methods	Sleep with the head elevated in 10–20 cm	Avoid nocturnal hypertension
		Reduces nocturnal natriuresis
		Activates the renin- angiotensin system
	Physical countermanouvres: squat, leg crossing, toe raising, bending at the waist, thigh contraction	Increment of orthostatic tolerance
	Support garments: leg stockings combined with abdominal binder	Reduces venous capacitance

TABLE 4.2 Pharmacological treatment of OH

Drugs	Action sympathomimetics	Doses daily	Main considerations	Side effects
Midodrine	Alpha 1 agonist	10–40 mg oral	Action onset: 0.5–1 h after ingestion	Paresthesias, piloerection, scalp itching or tingling, urinary urgency or retention
			Duration: 2–4 h. Risk of supine hypertension, last dose at 17 h	Supine hypertension
Pyridostigmine	Anticholinergic, increase sympathetic outflow at sympathetic ganglia	30–60 mg		Abdominal cramps, diarrhea, nausea, increased salivation, urinary urgency, bradycardia
Droxidopa (L-DOPS)	DOPS is converted to norepinephrine	100–600 mg TID	Action onset: 1 h after administration	Supine hypertension
			Duration: 6 h while standing	

(continued)

TABLE 4.2 (continued)

Drugs	Action sympathomimetics	Doses daily	Main considerations	Side effects
Volume expanders				
Fludrocortisone	Mineralocorticoid increase volume due to sodium retention	0.1–0.4 mg oral	Plasma half life is 2–3 h long-lasting effect Pressor action occurs after 1–2 weeks Not use in patients with congestive heart failure	Supine hypertension, ankle edema, hypokalemia, hypomagnesaemia, headache Reduce action of warfarin
Erythropoietin	Increase blood pressure treat the normocytic, normochromic anemia of autonomic failure	25–75 U/kg SQ	Dose given 3 times a week until to get a normal hematocrit level Need iron supplementation	Supine hypertension
Desmopressin	Vasopressin analogue	5–40 μg nasal spray	Single dose, potent effect	Water intoxication, hyponatremia
Prevent vasodilatation				
Octeotride	Somatostatin analogue Inhibits vasodilators Gastrointestinal peptides	25–200 μg	To prevent postprandial hypotension	Abdominal cramps. nausea, chronic use: hyperglycemia, risk of gallstones

Table 4.3 Treatment of GI dysfunction

Treatment	Non-pharmacogical	Pharmacological	Doses daily	Side effects
Constipation				
	Diet: fiber supplementation, 15 g/day	Mild laxatives:		Chronic use:
	Training of defecation habit	Magnesium salts	2–4 tablets	Electrolytes loss
	Adequate liquid ingestion for prevention of intestinal	Polyethylene glycol	17 g in 25 mL 1 or 2	
	Obstruction	Lactulose	15–30 mL TID	Colonic morphological changes
	Surgery for intractable colonic inertia	Bulk agent: psyllium	1 tsp to 3	
		Stool softeners: docusate	100 mg BID	

(continued)

Table 4.3 (continued)

Treatment	Non-pharmacogical	Pharmacological	Doses daily	Side effects
		Chloride channel action:		
		Lubiprostone	24 mcg twice	
		Pyridostigmine	180–540 mg	Nausea, vomiting, diarrhea
		Cathartics: Bisacodyl	10 mg up 3 times a week	
		Antibiotics to prevent		
		Bacterial overgrowth	7–10 days every month	
Gastroparesia Nutritional support: low fat, low fiber oral				
	Supplementation via jejunal feeding tube	Metoclopramide	5–20 mg 4 times	Extrapiramidal signs
	Gastric stimulator (electrical)			Hyperprolactinemia
		Domperidone	10–30 mg 4 times	May prolonged QT interval

Symptom	Treatment	Dose	Side effects
	Erythromycin	50–250 mg 4 times	Fatal arrhythmias (used with CYP3A inhibitors)
	Pyridostigmine	180–540 mg	Nausea, vomiting, diarrhea
	Bethanecol	25 mg 4 times	
	Pyloric botulinum toxin	Endoscopic injection	
Dysphagia	Speech therapy, swallowing training		
	feeding tube, gastroscopic		
Excessive drooling	Anticholinergic:		Constipation, urinary retention, confusion, blurred vision
	Glycopyrrolate	0.5–2 mg	
	Scopolamine transderm	1.5 mg patch	
	Botulinum toxin	Intraglandular injection	

TABLE 4.4 Management of genito-urinary dysfunction

Treatment	Non pharmacological	Pharmacological	Doses daily PO (mg)	Side effects
Storage dysfunction	Education: Timetable of micturition voiding frequency, and learn to hold urine, pelvic floor exercises	Antimuscarinics:		Dry mouth, constipation, blurred vision risk of glaucoma, confusion, risk of glaucoma, confusion, risk of increase post void urine residual
		Oxybutinin	2.5–20	
		Tolterodine	4	
	Reduction of liquid ingestion:1–2 L daily	Propantheline	45–90	
		Trospium	40	
	Surgical treatment: detrusor myectomy for overactive bladder	Imipramine	15–50	
		Darifenacin	7.5–15	
		Solifenacin	5–10	

	Adjunt Desmopressin	0.1–0.2	Allergic reaction, hyponatremia
	Antimuscarinics applied intravesical		Less side effects
	Botulinum injection in the bladder intravesical drugs acting on TRPV1 receptors		Allergic reactions, muscle weakness away from the injection
Voiding dysfunction	Learn about risk of urinary infections		
	Clean intermittent self or third-party catheterization		
	Botulinum injection in the external sphincter for spasticity		Allergic reactions, muscle weakness away from the injection
	Intravesical electro stimulation, useful in peripheral lesions with preserved detrusor activity		
	Alfa blockers to decrease		Risk of worsening OH, stomach pain

(continued)

TABLE 4.4 (Continued)

Treatment	Non pharmacological	Pharmacological	Doses daily	Side effects
		Bladder outlet resistance:		Drug interaction: PDE 5 inhibitors
		Terazocin	1–10	Antibiotics and HIV medication
		Doxazocin	1–8	Antidepressants
Erectile dysfunction	Psychological therapy	PDE 5 inhibitors:		
	Life style: physical activity, habits vacuum pump device	Sildenafil	25–100	Headache, blue vision, ischemic optic
		Tadalafil	5–20	Neuropathy, increase OH, interaction with drugs for fungal and HIV infection
		Vardenafil	2.5–20	
		Intracavernous drugs		Penile pain and edema and hematoma
		Alprostadil, Papaverine		Penile nodules or plaques, Priapism

Part II
Clinical Cases

Chapter 5
Acute or Subacute Pure Generalized Autonomic Failure

Juan Idiaquez, Eduardo Benarroch, and Martin Nogues

5.1 Case 1 Autoimmune Autonomic Ganglionopathy (AAG)

A 44-year-old man presented for evaluation due to progressive symptoms of orthostatic intolerance, including dizziness and lightheadedness on standing over the past 3 weeks. He had several episodes of syncope that rendered him unable to work. Concurrently, he noticed abdominal bloating, constipation, dry mouth, nycturia, erectile dysfunction, and intolerance to bright light. General examination was normal. Supine blood pressure was 130/67 mmHg; on standing blood pressure

J. Idiaquez (✉)
Universidad de Valparaiso, Viña del Mar, Chile
e-mail: idiaquez@123.cl

E. Benarroch
Mayo Clinic, Rochester, MN, USA
e-mail: benarroch@mayo.edu

M. Nogues
Clinica Fleni, Buenos Aires, Argentina
e-mail: mnogues@fleni.org.ar

© Springer International Publishing AG 2018   45
J. Idiaquez et al. (eds.), *Evaluation and Management of Autonomic Disorders*,
https://doi.org/10.1007/978-3-319-72251-1_5

dropped to 60/35 mmHg, without change in heart rate (supine, 74 bpm; standing, 75 bpm). Supine plasma noradrenaline levels were 10 pg/mL; levels upon standing were 60 pg/mL. Neurological examination showed normal mental status; cranial nerve examination showed bilateral mydriasis without oculomotor abnormalities. Muscle tone, strength, and deep tendon reflexes were normal. Sensory examination was normal. Autonomic testing confirmed the presence of severe orthostatic hypotension. Beat-to-beat blood pressure responses during the Valsalva maneuver showed a lack of recovery during late phase II and absent overshoot during phase IV. Heart rate responses to deep breathing and Valsalva ratio were severely reduced, indicating cardiovagal denervation. There was evidence of parasympathetic denervation of the pupils, which were reactive to diluted pilocarpine 0.00625%, due to denervation supersensitivity.

5.2   Questions for Consideration

1. **What was the differential diagnosis suggested by clinical evaluation and autonomic testing?**
   The presence of subacute generalized autonomic dysfunction with prominent orthostatic hypotension includes the following diagnoses:

A. **Paraneoplastic autonomic neuropathy**: there is a presentation of a subacute widespread sympathetic and parasympathetic dysfunction, including neurogenic orthostatic hypotension with severe disabling orthostatic intolerance and syncope; gastrointestinal symptoms mainly constipation, urinary retention, erectile dysfunction, and dry eyes and mouth; and difficulty in vision in bright light due to pupillary dysfunction. Often it is associated with a peripheral motor or sensory polyneuropathy or ganglionopathy or with central nervous system dysfunction.

B. **Autoimmune autonomic ganglionopathy (AAG):** the patient develops a subacute prominent orthostatic hypotension, gastrointestinal symptoms, and urinary, sudomotor, and erectile dysfunction. Pupillary denervation present with bilateral mydriasis. In addition, a sicca syndrome may be present.

Our patient's symptoms and signs were only related to autonomic manifestations, his general examination was normal, and his neurological examination showed cognitive, motor, and sensory examination.

2. **Which investigations were useful to distinguish among possible diagnosis?**

Nerve conduction and EMG studies were normal. CT of the chest/abdomen/pelvis were normal. Testicular ultrasonography was normal. Antibodies SSA and SSB were negative. Paraneoplastic: Antineuronal nuclear antibody type 1 (ANNA-1, (anti Hu) and type 2 (anti Ri), Purkinje cell cytoplasmic antibody type 2 (PCA-2), amphiphysin antibody, and collapsing response-mediator protein 5 (CRMP-5) were all negatives. Serum anti-ganglionic acetylcholine receptor antibodies (α3 nAChR) showed high titer: 3.6 nmol/L (normal <0.05).

3. **What was the most likely diagnosis?**

Electrophysiological tests did not show motor or sensory peripheral nerve involvement; the normal imaging studies and negative paraneoplastic antibody titers argued against a paraneoplastic autonomic neuropathy.

High titers of ganglionic acetylcholine receptor (α3 nAChR) antibodies support the diagnosis of AAG.

4. **How was the patient treated?**

Orthostatic hypotension was treated with a combination of fludrocortisone, midodrine, and pyridostigmine (see Tables 4.1 and 4.2). He also received immunomodulatory therapy with intravenous immunoglobulin 0.4 g/kg daily for 5 days followed by 0.4 g/kg weekly for 6 weeks as well as a tapering course of oral prednisone and azathioprine for 2 years. The patient improved gradually. Three-year follow-up showed improvement of gastrointestinal and sudomotor symptoms, but moderate orthostatic intolerance persisted. During that period, repeated imaging studies did not reveal a systemic cancer.

5.3 Discussion

The typical clinical picture of AAG includes severe OH with pupillary dysfunction and gastrointestinal, sudomotor, and genitourinary dysfunction.

The present case showed generalized autonomic manifestations without cognitive, motor, or sensory dysfunction. High AChR antibodies were associated with a severe autonomic dysfunction. Regarding autonomic ganglionopathy associated with a malignant tumor, our patient did not show paraneoplastic autoantibody titers, and imaging did not show malignancies. It is known that patients with paraneoplastic neuropathy may not show a tumor at the time of the diagnosis. A follow-up of the patient for at least 3 years, with periodical screening tests for neoplasia, is required. Small-cell lung carcinoma (SLC), thymoma, lymphomas, and adenocarcinomas are the main associated tumors.

We followed up the patient for 6 years and no evidence for neoplasia was found.

Paraneoplastic autonomic neuropathy often coexists with other paraneoplastic syndromes such as sensory and motor ganglionopathy, axonal polyneuropathy, or limbic encephalitis.

Other autoimmune disorders affecting the autonomic nervous system are Sjögren syndrome and Lambert-Eaton syndrome; both conditions present with neuromuscular deficits.

Our patient did not show symptoms or signs of motor or sensory peripheral polyneuropathy.

5.4 Relevant Aspect of AAG

Etiology: In 2000, Vernino et al. established AAG as an acquired immune-mediated autonomic disorder, before there were several clinical case reports of pure pandysautonomia, acute pandysautonomia, and idiopathic autonomic neuropathy. There is strong evidence that AAG is an autoimmune disorder, based upon animal models: passive transfer of ACh antibodies and immunization against ACh antibodies produce a similar disorder to human AAG.

Clinical manifestations: This immune-mediated disorder is characterized by a generalized and varied spectrum of autonomic dysfunction. Antecedent of a previous viral infection has been reported. The onset may be acute, subacute, or gradual. The classical presentation is subacute with a monophasic course. It occurs in adult life, and patients develop orthostatic hypotension and gastrointestinal, urinary, sudomotor, erectile, and pupillary dysfunction. Orthostatic intolerance may be severe; among common gastrointestinal symptoms are nausea, vomiting, early satiety, bloating, and constipation; some patients may present with achalasia and paralytic ileus. Sudomotor dysfunction in the majority of patients is characterized by a widespread postganglionic sudomotor dysfunction; a distal pattern of anhidrosis occurs in a minority of patients. Pupillary dysfunction present with bilateral mydriasis reflecting parasympathetic denervation is a prominent sign in AAG. A sympathetic and mixed denervation of the pupils can occur.

There is a chronic AAG phenotype with a slowly progressive autonomic dysfunction; there are no relevant differences in autonomic symptom severity, titers of ganglionic AChR antibodies, and response to treatment between the subacute and chronic phenotypes. The insidious presentation of chronic AAG may resemble pure autonomic failure (PAF), a neurodegenerative α-synucleinopathy, with compromise of the autonomic ganglion cells and their postganglionic axons.

Some patients may present with extra autonomic manifestations: minor sensory symptoms without objective clinical signs, coughing episodes, psychiatric symptoms, reversible cognitive deficits, encephalopathy co-occurring with AAG, inappropriate secretion of antidiuretic hormone, hyponatremia, and amenorrhea.

Diagnosis: In AAG, antibodies to the ganglionic AChR are present in about 50% of the patients with the clinical picture of widespread sympathetic and parasympathetic dysfunction. There is a direct relationship between the severity of autonomic dysfunction and high AChR antibody titers. Some patients with seronegative AAG may respond to immunomodulation. Possibly other still unidentified antibodies are responsible. A minority of patients with seronegative AAG may convert to a paraneoplastic form during the follow-up.

Antibodies specific for ganglionic AChR may be variable positive in conditions other than AAG like paraneoplastic AAG, thymoma, Lambert-Eaton syndrome, some cases of postural tachycardia syndrome, and some focal and restricted autonomic neuropathies (chronic idiopathic anhidrosis, idiopathic gastrointestinal dysmotility, acute cholinergic neuropathy, and acute sympathetic neuropathy). The antibody titers in such conditions are lower than those seen in typical AAG, and their clinical significance is uncertain.

5.5   Treatment and Prognosis

Acute treatment alternatives:

1. Intravenous immunoglobulin: a dose of 0.4 g/kg daily for 3 to 5 consecutive days.
2. Intravenous methylprednisolone: 1 g daily for 3 to 5 consecutive days. Both therapies must be followed by a weekly dose for 6 to 12 weeks.
3. Plasma exchange may be used after the immunoglobulin administration if the symptoms persist.

Chronic therapy alternatives:

1. Oral prednisone: 1 mg/kg daily. Long-term use of steroids is associated with different adverse events including diabetes, infections, hypertension, osteoporosis, and psychiatric disorders.
2. Azathioprine: 100 mg per day for 2 months; adverse events of azathioprine include nausea, vomiting, rash, hepatotoxicity, pancreatitis, and leukopenia. Also, a malignant tumor is a potential complication.
3. Mycophenolate mofetil 1 mg twice daily; adverse events include nausea, abdominal pain, diarrhea, drug-induced fever, and leucopenia.

There are reports of therapy with rituximab; a combined immunosuppressive therapy may be useful in some patients.

Immunotherapy may produce a complete or a partial recovery. There is a chronic form of AAG with persistent autonomic symptoms during life. A spontaneous incomplete recover can occur in about one-third of patients.

5.6 Key Points

Acute or subacute generalized autonomic dysfunction with sparing of the somatic motor and sensory functions may be a treatable condition.

Paraneoplastic autonomic neuropathy may present with a similar clinical picture of AAG. In paraneoplastic conditions, there is coexistence of different peripheral and central nervous system syndromes.

Clinical and laboratory testing must be focused on autoimmune studies (including paraneoplastic antibodies) and detection of a malignant tumor.

In about 50% of AAG patients, elevated antibodies to the ganglionic AChR are present, and antibody titers level correlates with the severity of the autonomic dysfunction.

Immunomodulation and immunosuppressive drugs are useful to treat AAG. Early therapeutic intervention before neuronal cell loss occurs is crucial.

In AAG, spontaneous recovery may occur. Immunotherapy may produce a complete or a partial recovery. There is a chronic form of AAG with persistent autonomic symptoms during life.

Bibliography

1. Vernino S, Low PA, Fealey RD, Stewart JD, Farrugia G, Lennon VA. Autoantibodies to ganglionic acetylcholine receptors in autoimmune autonomic neuropathies. N Engl J Med. 2000;343:847–55.
2. Gibbons CH, Vernino SA, Freeman R. Combined immunomodulatory therapy in autoimmune autonomic ganglionopathy. Arch Neurol. 2008;65:213–7.
3. Koike H, Wanatabe H, Sobue G. The spectrum of immune-mediated autonomic neuropathies: insights from the clinicopathological features. J Neurol Neurosurg Psychiatry. 2013;84:98–106.

4. Winston N, Vernino S. Recent advances in autoimmune autonomic ganglionopathy. Curr Opin Neurol. 2010;23:514–8.
5. Gibbons CH, Vernino SA, Freeman R. Combined immunomodulatory therapy in autoimmune autonomic ganglionopathy. Arch Neurol. 2008;65(2):213–7.
6. Iodice V, Sandroni P. Autonomic neuropathies. Continuum (Minneap Minn). 2014;20((5 Peripheral Nervous System Disorders)):1373–97.

Chapter 6
Pure Autonomic Failure

Juan Idiaquez, Eduardo Benarroch, and Martin Nogues

6.1 Case 1. Pure Autonomic Failure (PAF)

A 62-year-old man is evaluated for slowly progressive autonomic symptoms suffered for about 15 years. He first complained of erectile dysfunction and progressive orthostatic intolerance, including faintness, fatigue, and leg weakness while walking. He also had several episodes of syncope, 5 years ago the syncopal episodes became frequent, and orthostatic hypotension was found. He also noticed urinary urgency and diminished sweating. Neither he nor his wife noticed any sleep disturbance. General examination was normal. Supine blood pressure was 197/101 mmHg, on standing with heart rate of 65 bpm; standing blood pressure dropped to 90/52 mmHg, without compensatory heart rate to 72 bpm. Neurological examination showed normal mental status.

J. Idiaquez (✉)
Universidad de Valparaiso, Viña del Mar, Chile
e-mail: idiaquez@123.cl

E. Benarroch
Mayo Clinic, Rochester, MN, USA
e-mail: benarroch@mayo.edu

M. Nogues
Clinica Fleni, Buenos Aires, Argentina
e-mail: mnogues@fleni.org.ar

© Springer International Publishing AG 2018
J. Idiaquez et al. (eds.), *Evaluation and Management of Autonomic Disorders*,
https://doi.org/10.1007/978-3-319-72251-1_6

Cranial nerves examination showed symmetric reactive pupils and normal oculomotor function. Motor examination showed normal gait, strength, and muscle tone with the absence of pyramidal, extrapyramidal, and cerebellar signs. Sensation was normal.

Autonomic testing showed severe orthostatic hypotension. Supine plasma norepinephrine was low (70 pg/mL) and did not increase significantly on standing (92 pg/mL). Valsalva maneuver showed impaired blood pressure recovery during late phase II and IV. There were reduced heart rate changes in response to deep breathing, indicating of cardiovagal denervation. Sympathetic skin responses were absent in the soles. Motor and sensory peripheral nerve conductions were normal.

Ambulatory blood pressure monitoring showed nocturnal hypertension. Brain MRI (with T2 signal) and peripheral nerve conduction studies were normal.

6.2   Questions for Consideration

1. **What is the differential diagnosis based on clinical evaluation and autonomic testing?**
   The presence of slowly progressive autonomic failure with severe orthostatic hypotension and without neurological signs of central nervous system compromise includes the following diagnoses:

   A. **Chronic variant of autoimmune autonomic ganglionopathy (AAG):** A small group of patients with AAG develop slowly progressive orthostatic hypotension with prominent orthostatic intolerance and gastrointestinal, genitourinary, pupil, and sudomotor dysfunction. Also, dry eyes and mouth occur. These patients do not show any peripheral or central nervous system signs. Our patient's symptoms were only related to autonomic manifestations, his general examination was normal, and his neurological examination showed normal cognitive, cranial nerves (including pupils) motor, and sensory examination.

B. **Autonomic failure as initial presentation of a synucle-inopathy**: Multiple system atrophy (MSA), Parkinson's disease (PD), and dementia with Lewy bodies (DLB) may present with early autonomic failure for several years before the complete phenotype of the synucle-inopathy develops. These cases are initially diagnosed as "pure" autonomic failure (PAF). In MSA, PD, and DLB, the presence of rapid eye movement (REM) sleep behavior disorder (RBD) is characteristic. The time of conversion from a PAF phenotype to a MSA, PD, or DLB phenotype is variable, about one third of patients, and conversion occurs in 5 years.

Our patient did not notice sleep disturbances, and the follow-up during 8 years did not show Parkinsonism, cerebellar, or pyramidal signs.

2. **Which clinical criteria and tests were useful to support the possible diagnosis?**
The clinical involvement limited to autonomic manifestations during a follow-up period of 8 years and past history of autonomic symptoms for about 15 years without development of Parkinsonism, cerebellar ataxia, or dementia would be consistent with PAF. The presence of orthostatic hypotension accompanied with anhidrosis, without severe bladder dysfunction and normal pupillary function, would be consistent with this diagnosis. The finding of a remarkable low supine plasma norepinephrine without significant increase on standing and negative titer of serum anti-ganglionic acetylcholine receptor antibodies ($\alpha 3$ nAChR) supports this diagnosis.

3. **What was the most likely diagnosis?**
Long-standing autonomic failure, without evidence of central neurodegeneration, is compatible with PAF.

4. **How was the patient treated?**
Orthostatic hypotension was treated with non-pharmacological approaches (see Table 4.1) and a combination of fludrocortisone, midodrine, and pyridostigmine (see Table 4.2).

6.3   Discussion

The present case showed long-term generalized autonomic manifestations without cognitive, motor, or sensory dysfunction. Low circulating NE without increment on standing indicates that the patient had a disease that compromises postganglionic autonomic neurons. Chronic AAG may present with similar clinical pattern, but our patient did not show pupillary dysfunction, which is very common in this disorder, and had no detectable ganglionic AChR antibodies. Whereas a seronegative chronic variant of AAG cannot be excluded, the temporal profile of autonomic failure suggests a degenerative rather than an autoimmune cause. A follow-up of the patient for at least 8 years, without conversion to MSA, PD, or LBD, would support the clinical diagnosis of PAF. Consistent with PAF, bladder symptoms were only moderate in our patient. In MSA patients when orthostatic hypotension is the initial manifestation, the presence of motor signs and severe bladder dysfunction occurs promptly. The presence of autonomic failure with RBD is suggestive of a synucleinopathy with compromise of brainstem; our patient did not show symptoms compatible with RBD.

6.4   Relevant Aspect of PAF

Etiology: PAF is a sporadic disorder characterized by slowly progressive neurogenic orthostatic hypotension accompanied by sudomotor, urogenital, and gastrointestinal symptoms; pathological studies showed degeneration restricted to peripheral autonomic neurons, with accumulation of α synuclein in Lewy bodies within sympathetic ganglia and Lewy neurites through sympathetic axons in the heart, bladder, periadrenal tissue, colon, and skin. The presence of α synuclein restricted to peripheral autonomic neurons and the knowledge that some patients with PAF convert to a central nervous system compromise support the notion that PAF is a phenotype of synucleinopathy.

Clinical manifestations: The typical onset is between 50 and 70 years of age. Autonomic symptoms are insidious so that in early stage of the disease, slowly progressive symptoms of orthostatic intolerance are not detected until a severe orthostatic hypotension with repeated syncope occurs. Also the patient complains diminished sweating and intolerance to hot environment. Mild to moderate symptoms of urgency and augmented frequency of micturition appears after several years of evolution. Urinary incontinence is less frequent. Erectile and ejaculatory dysfunction may be present. Constipation occurs in the majority of patients; it may be an early or later manifestation. Other gastrointestinal symptoms are rare.

Diagnosis: PAF must be considered as an initial presumptive clinical diagnosis. The long-term follow-up for period of 5 years of isolated autonomic failure without motor manifestations is the only useful criteria to support the diagnosis.

6.5 Treatment and Prognosis

There is no disease-specific treatment. Management of OH, constipation, and urinary dysfunction is described in the corresponding chapters. In PAF, there is a slowly progressive deterioration of autonomic functions, and the prognosis is benign so patients may survive for decades.

6.6 Key Points

1. PAF is a clinical diagnosis based on long-term presence of autonomic dysfunction without development of motor signs.
2. A group of patients with the initial diagnosis of PAF evolve to MSA, PD, or LBD within a variable period of up to 10 years, typically 4–5 years.
3. The presence of slowly progressive orthostatic symptoms accompanied with reduced sweating, without severe gas-

trointestinal and bladder dysfunction, suggests a PAF phenotype.
4. Predictors of conversion of PAF phenotype to MSA, PD, or LBD are normal plasma NE, the presence of early bladder dysfunction, and early occurrence of RBD.

Bibliography

1. Mabuchi N, Hirayama M, Koike Y, Watanabe H, Ito H, Kobayashi R, Hamada K, Sobue G. Progression and prognosis in pure autonomic failure (PAF): comparison with multiple system atrophy. J Neurol Neurosurg Psychiatry. 2005;76:947–52.
2. Kaufmann H, Norcliffe-Kaufmann L, Palma JA, Biaggioni I, Low PA, Singer W, Goldstein DS, Peltier AC, Shibao CA, Gibbons CH, Freeman R, Robertson D. Autonomic disorders consortium. Natural history of pure autonomic failure: a United States prospective cohort. Ann Neurol. 2017;81(2):287–97.
3. Singer W, Berini SE, Sandroni P, Fealey RD, Coon EA, Suarez MD, Benarroch EE, Low PA. Pure autonomic failure: predictors of conversion to clinical CNS involvement. Neurology. 2017;88(12):1129–36.

Chapter 7

Chronic Autonomic Failure Associated with Parkinsonism, Ataxia or Dementia

Juan Idiaquez, Eduardo Benarroch, and Martin Nogues

Abstract Clinical case. Differential diagnosis: Synucleinopathies with parkinsonism (PD, MSA, DLB). Diagnosis: Temporal profile of motor and autonomic dysfunction, brain MRI, cardiac sympathetic imaging. Main autonomic manifestations of PD: orthostatic hypotension, gastrointestinal, bladder dysfunction and sudomotor dysfunction. Symptoms management and prognosis.

J. Idiaquez (✉)
Universidad de Valparaiso, Viña del Mar, Chile
e-mail: idiaquez@123.cl

E. Benarroch
Mayo Clinic, Rochester, MN, USA
e-mail: benarroch@mayo.edu

M. Nogues
Clinica Fleni, Buenos Aires, Argentina
e-mail: mnogues@fleni.org.ar

7.1   Case 1. Parkinson's Disease

A 70-year-old man referred for evaluation of mild orthostatic intolerance and postprandial dizziness over 1-year duration. He also noticed constipation, urinary urgency, and nocturia. He did not complain of sweating disturbance. His wife reported that the patient exhibited violent movements and vocalizations during sleep, as he was enacting his dreams. General examination was normal. Neurological examination showed normal mental status. Cranial nerve examination showed anosmia. Pupil diameter and reactivity and eye movements were normal. Motor examination reduced left arm swing and resting tremor and cogwheel rigidity in the left upper limb. There were no pyramidal and cerebellar signs. Sensation was normal. Autonomic testing showed orthostatic hypotension (OH). Supine blood pressure was 130/63 mmHg; on standing it dropped to 109/51 mmHg, and heart rate increased (supine, 60 bpm; standing, 72 bpm). Supine norepinephrine was reduced to 80 pg/mL but increased upon standing (156 pg/mL). Valsalva maneuver showed an abnormal recovery of blood pressure during late phase II. Cardiovagal testing showed reduced heart rate responses to deep breathing. Sympathetic skin responses were normal. Ambulatory blood pressure monitoring showed nocturnal hypertension. History excluded secondary causes of Parkinsonism such as drugs, toxins, stroke, or head trauma. A follow-up during 5 years showed a slowly progressive motor deterioration, with bradykinesia and bilateral tremor. Mental status remains normal.

7.2   Questions for Consideration

1. **What was the differential diagnosis suggested by clinical evaluation and autonomic testing?**
   The presence of Parkinsonian signs with autonomic failure includes the following diagnoses:

A. **Multiple system atrophy with predominant Parkinsonism (MSA-P):** These patients present with a rapidly progressive Parkinsonism nonresponsive to levodopa and severe autonomic dysfunction: incapacitating orthostatic hypotension, severe urinary manifestations including urgency, retardation in initiating urination and urge incontinence, and loss of sweating. In many cases, inspiratory gasps and stridor are present.

Our patient had slowly progressive Parkinsonism that responded to levodopa, with non-disabling autonomic dysfunction and without respiratory signs.

B. **Dementia with Lewy bodies** (DLB) present with a progressive fluctuating cognitive decline, Parkinsonism, and autonomic failure. Cognitive dysfunction occurs within the first year of the motor signs and is often accompanied with visual hallucinations. The most common symptoms are orthostatic hypotension, incontinence, and constipation.

Our patient did not show cognitive dysfunction during long-term follow-up.

2. **Which clinical criteria and tests may be useful to support the possible diagnosis?**

The presence of Parkinsonism that responds to levodopa, preserved cognitive function, and mild autonomic failure suggests the diagnosis of Parkinson disease (PD) with autonomic failure. The brain MRI did not show abnormal signals. When available, cardiac imaging using MIBG (123-meta-iodobenzylguanidine) shows evidence of cardiac sympathetic denervation. The low values of supine norepinephrine in plasma may support the presence of peripheral sympathetic denervation.

3. **What was the most likely diagnosis?**

Parkinson's disease (PD).

4. **How was the patient treated**?

There was good response of motor signs to levodopa. Orthostatic hypotension was treated (see Tables 4.1 and 4.2) with a combination of fludrocortisone and midodrine.

7.3   Discussion

In this patient, the presence of slowly progressive asymmetric parkinsonian signs, accompanied with moderate autonomic failure, supports the clinical diagnosis of PD. In MSA, orthostatic hypotension and urinary dysfunction progress more rapidly to an incapacitating condition. During 5 years of follow-up, our patient did not present cognitive decline, so we can exclude a clinical diagnosis of DLB. Peripheral sympathetic denervation reflected by low circulating norepinephrine and by reduced cardiac MIBG uptake supports the clinical diagnosis of PD. In general, MSA typically show normal plasmatic norepinephrine and normal cardiac sympathetic innervation. However, some MSA cases may also have abnormal MIBG uptake.

7.4   Relevant Aspect of Autonomic Dysfunction in PD

Etiology: PD is a disorder with widespread α-synuclein pathology with loss of dopaminergic neurons of the substantia nigra, with α-synuclein accumulation in the soma (Lewy bodies) and fibrils of α-synuclein (Lewy neurites) in the axons. Deposits of α-synuclein are present in cerebral cortex, limbic system, nucleus basalis of Meynert, dorsal motor nucleus of the vagus nerve, sympathetic ganglia, and myenteric and mucosal plexus of the digestive tract.

7.5   Clinical Manifestations

1. Orthostatic hypotension
   The prevalence is about 30%, and their presence is associated with long-term evolution and treatment with dopaminergic agonists. In a subgroup of patients, OH can occur early in the disease, in some cases prior motor manifestations. Symptoms of orthostatic intolerance may show a dif-

ferent degree of severity, from asymptomatic OH that can give symptoms only in the presence of aggravating factors (dehydration, hypotensive drugs) to disabling OH with frequent falls. Postprandial hypotension and supine hypertension coexist with OH. Supine hypertension may increase the risk of cardiovascular diseases. During the disease progression, OH may contribute to cognitive decline. Transient worsening of working memory, executive, and visuospatial functions can occur on standing position. Twenty-four-hour ambulatory blood pressure monitoring, with a detailed patient report of symptoms, is a useful tool.

2. Gastrointestinal symptoms

   Constipation is the most relevant symptom, reported in 80–90% of patients, and may occur several years before motor manifestations. Drug treatment with anticholinergic and dopamine agonists may aggravate constipation. Megacolon and intestinal pseudo-obstruction can occur. PD patients may also complain straining of defecation. Dysphagia occurs late during progression of PD but occasionally may occur early; it is reported in 30–80% of patients. Aspiration (inhalation of liquid or food) is a potential complication of upper respiratory tract infections and pneumonia. Videofluoroscopy may show oropharyngeal and esophageal dysphagia in asymptomatic patients. Drooling of saliva occurs in 10–80% of patients, and it is associated with the presence of dysphagia; dysarthria and facial hypomimia are common associated features. However salivary production is reduced in PD, so patients may complain of dry mouth. Upper gastrointestinal symptoms, including nausea, vomiting, early satiety, and weight loss, are caused by gastroparesis. Standard meal labeled emptying studies show delayed gastric emptying of solid food in 90% of patients. Gastroparesis may be asymptomatic, but its presence may delay arrival of levodopa to intestine.

3. Urogenital symptoms

   Nocturia is reported in >60%, urinary urgency in 30–50%, augmented day time urinary frequency in 16–36%, and incontinence associated to urgency in 25% of PD patients. Urodynamic studies show detrusor overactivity and uninhibited external sphincter relaxation. Augmented post-residual micturition is not seen in PD. Loss of libido, erectile dysfunction, and hypersexuality related to dopaminergic agonist.

4. Sudomotor dysfunction

   Sweating symptoms vary from diminished sweating to hyperhidrosis, which occurs in off periods and dyskinesia. Quantification of sweating (QSART method) shows a percentage of anhidrosis in PD lower than in MSA.

Diagnosis: The presence of autonomic failure in PD is shown by sympathetic and parasympathetic reflex tests which indicate the level and severity of dysfunction, but these tests cannot always differentiate between different synucleinopathies. In general, low supine plasma NE level and imaging studies showing reduced cardiac uptake of NE precursors indicate peripheral sympathetic denervation and support the diagnosis of PD. In most PD cases, cardiac MIBG is reduced in 80–90% and is not related to the presence of OH. However, cardiac sympathetic denervation is also present also in LBD and PAF. In some cases, it has been found in patients with MSA.

Treatment and prognosis: Non-pharmacological and pharmacological treatments of autonomic symptoms are described in Chap. 4 (Tables 4.1, 4.2, 4.3, and 4.4). OH is a significant prognostic factor for cognitive decline and mortality.

7.6   Key Points

Autonomic symptoms due to gastrointestinal, urinary, cardiovascular, and sudomotor dysfunction are frequent in PD.

OH, postprandial hypotension, and supine hypertension coexist in PD patients.

Subclinical OH may produce symptoms due to aggravating factors.

Constipation, orthostatic hypotension, and urinary symptoms may precede motor manifestations of PD.

Autonomic failure interferes with daily life activities and OH worsens cognitive decline.

Abstract Clinical case. Differential diagnosis: Synucleinopathies with parkinsonism (MSA, PD, DLB). Diagnosis: Temporal profile of motor, respiratory and autonomic dysfunction. Brain MRI, bladder ultrasonography, polysommography. Main autonomic manifestations of PD: orthostatic hypotension, bladder, erectile, sudomotor and erectile dysfunction. Nocturnal stridor and sleep apnea. Symptoms management and prognosis.

7.7   Case 2. Multiple System Atrophy

A 51-year-old man is evaluated for a 2-year history of progressive motor symptoms including slow movements and stiffness in the upper limbs. During last year he presented dizziness on standing and episodes of syncope. He also noticed urinary urgency and erectile dysfunction. According to his wife, over the past 5 years, he has experienced sleep episodes characterized by shouting, punching, and occasionally leaping out of bed, as if he was enacting dreams. A neurological evaluation found normal cognitive function. Cranial nerve examinations showed normal pupils and oculomotor function. Motor examination showed bilateral rigidity and bradykinesia, without tremor. No pyramidal and cerebellar signs were found. Sensation was normal. He was started on levodopa. Autonomic testing showed orthostatic hypotension (OH). Supine blood pressure was 160/71 mmHg; on standing it dropped to 70/46 mmHg, without compensatory increase in heart rate (supine, 80 bpm; standing, 88 bpm). Valsalva maneuver showed an abnormal blood pressure profile during phases II and IV. There was impaired heart rate response to deep breathing indicating cardiovagal denervation. Ambulatory blood pressure monitoring showed nocturnal hypertension supine norepinephrine was normal (220 pg/mL) but did not increase on standing (231 pg/mL).

One year after the initial evaluation, he developed urinary retention and incontinence requiring intermittent catheterization. His wife noticed that during sleep the patient showed fewer vocalizations and movements but he presented stridor, snoring, and episodes of breathing pauses. During the day, he had inspiratory gasps and noted cold hands. The patient showed progressive motor deterioration without response to levodopa.

7.8   Questions for Consideration

1. **What was the differential diagnosis suggested by clinical evaluation and autonomic testing?**
   The presence of bilateral parkinsonian signs with orthostatic hypotension and urinary dysfunction includes the following diagnoses:

   A. **Parkinson's disease with autonomic failure:** patients typically present a slowly progressive asymmetric bradykinesia, tremor, or both, typically responsive to levodopa. These motor symptoms may be accompanied with gastrointestinal, genitourinary, and orthostatic intolerance symptoms. In our patient, there was a rapid progression of symmetric bradykinesia and rigidity with poor response to levodopa. Orthostatic intolerance and urinary symptoms were severe. Also, our patient had inspiratory gasps, and polysomnography showed sleep stridor and obstructive sleep apnea.

   B. **Dementia with Lewy bodies** (DLB): patients tend to be over 60 years of age and present parkinsonism, cognitive dysfunction, visual hallucinations, and orthostatic hypotension. Our patient did not show cognitive decline, and autonomic symptoms were prominent.

2. **Which clinical criteria and tests were useful to support the possible diagnosis?**
   Atypical Parkinsonism and rapid progression of autonomic compromise, accompanied by daytime and noctur-

nal respiratory symptoms, are compatible with multiple system atrophy.

Autonomic tests showed severe OH, cardiovagal and sympathetic denervation (absent late phase II and phase IV during the Valsalva maneuver), and sudomotor dysfunction indicating a generalized autonomic failure. Measurement of urine residual volume by ultrasonography showed a post-micturition residue of 300 cm^3. The brain MRI showed mild nonspecific putaminal atrophy. Polysomnography showed several episodes of central and obstructive apnea and laryngeal stridor. Normal values of supine norepinephrine in plasma without rise on standing are consistent with a central cause of sympathetic failure. Cardiac imaging, MIBG (123-meta-iodobenzylguanidine) signal was normal.

3. **What was the most likely diagnosis?**
   Multiple system atrophy with predominant Parkinsonism (MSA-P).

4. **How was the patient treated?**
   Orthostatic hypotension was treated with a combination of fludrocortisone, midodrine, and pyridostigmine (see Tables 4.1 and 4.2). For bladder voiding dysfunction, intermittent catheterization was utilized. Continuous positive airway pressure therapy was used for the treatment of laryngeal stridor and sleep apnea.

7.9   Discussion

Our patient presents a rapid deterioration of motor and autonomic functions. The presence of incomplete bladder emptying that evolves in a short period to a severe urinary retention and the disabling symptoms of orthostatic intolerance are in favor of MSA. The presence of severe OH with normal value of supine norepinephrine, without increase on standing and preserved peripheral cardiac imaging sympathetic innervation, is compatible with a central sympathetic denervation. Our patient had respiratory signs including nocturnal stridor due to laryngeal dystonia and involuntary inspiratory gasps, which are rare in PD. A polysomnography confirmed the presence of sleep apnea and laryngeal stridor. In MSA, impaired automatic ventilation implicates compromise of the brainstem respiratory network, including the pre-Bötzinger complex and the medullary raphe, which may cause sudden death. The occurrence of cold hands, due to abnormalities of the microcirculation also, supports the diagnosis.

7.10   Relevant Aspect of Autonomic Dysfunction in MSA

Etiology: MSA is a sporadic, rapidly progressive, multisystem, neurodegenerative fatal disease. Both sexes were affected equally. The most frequent clinical phenotype is that of autonomic failures associated with Parkinsonism (MSA-P). In Japan the more frequent form is associated with cerebellar ataxia (MSA-C). This disorder is characterized by abnormal deposition of the protein alpha-synuclein primarily in oligodendrocytes (glial cytoplasmic inclusions), with the presence of neuronal loss in the striatum, substantia nigra pars compacta, pontine nuclei, inferior olivary nuclei, cerebellum, and premotor and autonomic nuclei.

7.11   Clinical Manifestations

1. Orthostatic hypotension
   Severe OH, defined as a fall of systolic BP of at least 30 mmHg or diastolic BP of at least 15 mmHg, is a major and frequent finding (75%). Symptoms of orthostatic intolerance are rapidly progressive and disabling. They tend to occur at early stages and may precede motor manifestations. Postprandial hypotension is also a frequent complication. Patients with MSA with initial clinical phenotype of pure autonomic failure (PAF) may evolve to a MSA phenotype within few years. In MSA patients, OH is associated

with supine hypertension. OH may contribute to cognitive dysfunction like attention, visuospatial, and frontal executive dysfunction which occurs in MSA. Neurochemical and cardiac imaging studies indicate that OH in MSA is mainly due to central denervation. Morphological studies show loss of premotor sympathoexcitatory neurons in the rostral ventrolateral medulla and preganglionic sympathetic neurons in the intermediolateral cell column.

2. Genitourinary dysfunction

Urinary dysfunction is more common and severe than in PD and often is an early manifestation. Symptoms of urinary dysfunction are frequent (83%), including urge incontinence (73%), nocturia (74%), difficulty of voiding (79%), and incomplete bladder emptying (48%). Urodynamic studies show increase post-void residual (over 100 ml) in most of the patients. The cystometry initially shows detrusor hyperreflexia; progressive dysfunction of detrusor muscle activity causes an atonic bladder. The sphincter EMG shows neurogenic changes. The neuropathological basis for these findings includes neuronal loss in the pontine micturition center, sacral preganglionic neurons, and Onuf's nucleus.

Erectile dysfunction occurs in almost 100% of males, and it is an early manifestation in about 40%. Some patients seek urological therapy before a neurological evaluation. The onset of erectile dysfunction may precede the onset of urinary symptoms and the onset of OH. Preserved erectile function would argue against the clinical diagnosis of MSA.

3. Sudomotor manifestations

Symptoms are progressive loss of sweating and intolerance to hot environments, but patients may not report these symptoms spontaneously, and thus they should be asked about them. The typical finding is a global pattern of anhidrosis in the thermoregulatory sweat test (TST). In MSA, the finding of anhidrosis in the TST and preserved sudomotor axon reflex responses are consistent with a preganglionic disorder. Repeated TST showed progressive sweating loss. Postganglionic sudomotor dysfunction may occur at late stage of the disease.

4. Gastrointestinal manifestations

Oropharyngeal dysphagia may interfere with nutrition. Dysphagia, combined with laryngeal paresis, may provoke tracheal aspiration. Symptoms of gastroparesis may occur; involvement of the dorsal motor nucleus of the vagus may contribute to impairment of upper gastrointestinal motility. Chronic constipation is frequent and can occur at early stage. It may be severe and may result in fecal impaction and overflow diarrhea. Constipation in MSA is caused by factors like reduced bowel motility, chronic rectal impaction, and bedridden. Fecal incontinence due to weak anal sphincter is a less common impediment.

7.12   Diagnosis

The constellation of clinical features is the main tool for the diagnosis of probable MSA. Criteria are predominantly focused on the motor manifestations. Autonomic failure is relevant and can be a premotor indicator. Sympathetic and parasympathetic reflex tests are useful to assess the level and severity of autonomic dysfunction. There are tests that help to support the diagnosis. Neurochemical tests may show normal plasma levels of norepinephrine and dihydroxyphenylglycol (DHPG). A typical MRI finding in MSA-P is a hyperintense rim in the posterior putamen and putaminal atrophy, but this is not sensitive for early diagnosis. Diffusion-weighted MRI may show increase T2 signal in the putamen. In MSA-C, there is abnormal T2 signal in the basis pontis associated with cerebellar atrophy. Fluorodeoxyglucose PET scanning may show hypometabolism in the putamen. In MSA, cardiac imaging show preserved peripheral sympathetic innervation, but some MSA patients may show reduced cardiac MIBG uptake. Polysomnography is a useful tool to detect the presence of nocturnal laryngeal stridor, which supports the clinical diagnosis of MSA. Nocturnal stridor may occur in all stages of the disease; as disease progress, diurnal stridor may be present.

7.13   Treatment and Prognosis

Identification and early therapy for symptoms associated with neurogenic bladder dysfunction, laryngeal stridor, and dysphagia are important to increase survival in MSA patients. Non-pharmacological and pharmacological treatments of autonomic symptoms are described in Chap. 4 (Tables 4.1, 4.2, 4.3, and 4.4). Median survival from symptom onset in MSA is 8–10 years, but the spectrum ranges from 4 to 15 years. Regarding survival, older age of onset and the presence of early autonomic dysfunction are bad prognostic factors. Early urinary catheterization need and presence of stridor have been linked to decreased survival.

7.14   Key Points

The diagnosis of probable MSA is based mainly on clinical motor, autonomic, and respiratory features.

Severe urological dysfunction occurs in MSA; detrusor muscle hypoactivity and urinary retention are characteristic urodynamic findings.

Polysomnography must be performed in every MSA patient to detect laryngeal stridor and sleep apneas.

Early therapy for symptoms associated with urinary dysfunction, laryngeal stridor, and dysphagia can improve survival in MSA patients.

Bibliography

1. Espay AJ, LeWitt PA, Hauser RA, Merola A, Masellis M, Lang AE. Neurogenic orthostatic hypotension and supine hypertension in Parkinson's disease and related synucleinopathies: prioritization of treatment targets. Lancet Neurol. 2016;15:954–66.
2. Fasano A, Visanji N, Liu LWC, Lang AE, Pfeiffer RF. Gastrointestinal dysfunction in Parkinson's disease. Lancet Neurol. 2015;14:625–39.

3. Goldstein DS. Dysautonomia in Parkinson disease. Compr Physiol. 2014;4:805–26.

4. Vichayanrat E, Low DA, Iodice V, Stuebner E, Hagen EM, Mathias CJ. Twenty-four-hour ambulatory blood pressure and heart rate profiles in diagnosing orthostatic hypotension in Parkinson's disease and multiple system atrophy. Eur J Neurol. 2017;24:90–7.

5. Sakakibara R, Tateno F, Nagao T, Yamamoto T, Uchiyama T, Yamanishi T, Yano M, Kishi M, Tsuyusaki Y, Aiba Y. Bladder function of patients with Parkinson's disease. Eur J Neurol. 2017;24:90–7.

6. Benarroch EE, Smithson IL, Low PA, Parisi JE. Depletion of catecholaminergic neurons of the rostral ventrolateral medulla in multiple systems atrophy with autonomic failure. Ann Neurol. 1998;43:156–63.

7. Benarroch EE, Schmeichel AM, Sandroni P, Low PA, Parisi JE. Involvement of vagal autonomic nuclei in multiple system atrophy and Lewy body disease. Neurology. 2006;66(3):378–83.

8. Ito T, Sakakibara R, Yasuda K, Yamamoto T, Uchiyama T, Liu Z, et al. Incomplete emptying and urinary retention in multiple-system atrophy: when does it occur and how do we manage it? Mov Disord. 2006;21:816–23.

9. Jecmenica-Lukic M, Poewe W, Tolosa E, Wenning GK. Premotor signs and symptoms of multiple system atrophy. Lancet Neurol. 2012;11:361–8.

10. Iodice V, Lipp A, Ahlskog JE, Sandroni P, Fealey RD, Parisi JE, Matsumoto JY, Benarroch EE, Kimpinski K, Singer W, Gehrking TL, Gehrking JA, Sletten DM, Schmeichel AM, Bower JH, Gilman S, Figueroa J, Low PA. Autopsy confirmed multiple system atrophy cases: Mayo experience and role of autonomic function tests. J Neurol Neurosurg Psychiatry. 2012;83:453–9.

11. Coon E, Sletten D, Suarez M, Mandrekar J, Ahlskog J, Bower J, Matsumoto J, Silber Benarroch E, Fealey R, Sandroni P, Low PA, Singer W. Clinical features and autonomic testing predict. Survival in multiple system atrophy. Brain. 2015;138:3623–31.

12. Coon EA, Fealey RD, Sletten DM, Mandrekar JN, Benarroch EE, Sandroni P, Low PA, Singer W. Anhidrosis in multiple system atrophy involves pre- and postganglionic sudomotor dysfunction. Mov Disord. 2017;32:397–404.

Chapter 8
Autonomic Failure in Chronic Peripheral Neuropathy

Juan Idiaquez, Eduardo Benarroch, and Martin Nogues

Abstract   Clinical case. Differential diagnosis: Diabetic neuropathy, Amyloidosis, uremic neuropathy, B12 vitamin deficiency, Paraneoplastic autonomic neuropathy, HIV infection, alcoholic neuropathy. Diagnosis: presence of peripheral polyneuropathy, specific blood tests. Main autonomic manifestations of diabetic neuropathy: cardiovascular autonomic neuropathy (CAN), bladder, gastrointestinal, sudomotor and erectile dysfunction. Symptoms management. CAN and survival prognosis.

J. Idiaquez (✉)
Universidad de Valparaiso, Viña del Mar, Chile
e-mail: idiaquez@123.cl

E. Benarroch
Mayo Clinic, Rochester, MN, USA
e-mail: benarroch@mayo.edu

M. Nogues
Clinica Fleni, Buenos Aires, Argentina
e-mail: mnogues@fleni.org.ar

© Springer International Publishing AG 2018   73
J. Idiaquez et al. (eds.), *Evaluation and Management of Autonomic Disorders*,
https://doi.org/10.1007/978-3-319-72251-1_8

8.1   Case 1. Diabetic Neuropathy

A 55-year-old man is referred for progressive fatigue, poly-
uria, and thirst and weight loss over the past 7 years. At that
time, a clinical evaluation showed hyperglycemia; he was
treated with an oral hypoglycemic drug that provoked episodes of hypoglycemia. Afterward the patient did not attend
regularly to periodic medical control. Four years ago, he
started noticing painful paresthesia in his feet. He then
started noticing mild gait unsteadiness. More recently, he had
several syncopal attacks, constipation, and nocturnal episodes
of diarrhea. He had difficulty to initiate micturition and erectile dysfunction with preserved sexual desire. He did not refer
any other medical condition and he denied alcohol or drug
consumption. He presented an acute febrile episode caused
by urinary tract infection. He was admitted to the hospital.
Blood test showed a fasting blood glucose of 230 mg/dL and
hemoglobin A1c of 7.9. Creatinine was normal. Urine sample
showed presence of pyuria and positive urinary culture
(*Escherichia coli*). He received antibiotic therapy. Neurological
evaluation showed normal cognitive status, Cranial nerve
examination was normal. Motor examination showed
unsteadiness on tandem walk and normal strength with
absent ankle jerks. He had loss of sensation for pinprick, temperature, light touch, and vibration on feet.

Autonomic testing showed orthostatic hypotension. Supine
blood pressure (BP) was 140/67 mmHg with a heart rate
(HR) of 80 bpm; on standing BP dropped to 100/50 mmHg,
with a HR of 88 bpm. Heart rate response to deep breathing
and Valsalva ratio were markedly reduced indicating severe
cardiovagal denervation. Blood pressure profile during the
Valsalva maneuver showed lack of BP recovery during late
phase II and lack of phase IV overshoot. Thermoregulatory
sweating test (iodine-starch) showed an area of symmetrical
anhidrosis in both feet and hands. Electrochemical skin con-
ductance (Sudoscan) was reduced in feet and hands. Nerve
conduction studies showed normal peroneal motor conduction velocities. Sural nerve amplitude was reduced.

8.2 Questions for Consideration

1. **What is the differential diagnosis suggested by clinical evaluation and autonomic testing?**

   A. **Diabetic neuropathy: The typical** phenotype is that of generalized sensorimotor polyneuropathy with autonomic dysfunction; there is a progressive compromise of both somatic and autonomic nerve fibers. Cardiovascular, genitourinary, gastrointestinal, and sudomotor dysfunction evolve from subclinical abnormalities to severe clinical manifestations.

   B. **Amyloidosis**: AL amyloidosis and transthyretin familial variety may present a generalized autonomic dysfunction, associated with a distal sensorimotor polyneuropathy; also autonomic manifestation can occur isolated.

   C. **Uremic neuropathy:** Patients present with a slowly progressive distal symmetrical polyneuropathy with distal paresthesia. Autonomic manifestations include orthostatic hypotension, gastrointestinal dysfunction, sudomotor dysfunction, and erectile dysfunction. Autonomic test may show cardiovascular and sudomotor dysfunction.

   D. **Vitamin B12 deficiency.** Patients may present neurological symptoms without hematological abnormalities. The neuropathy associated with vitamin B12 deficiency frequently begins with sensory symptoms in the feet. Patients may also show motor signs due to corticospinal tract involvement. Autonomic dysfunction is predominantly sympathetic with orthostatic hypotension and sudomotor dysfunction.

   E. **Paraneoplastic autonomic neuropathy**: There is a subacute or progressive onset of widespread autonomic dysfunction, including orthostatic hypotension, gastrointestinal symptoms, urinary retention, erectile dysfunction, and sicca syndrome. Frequently a sensorimotor polyneuropathy or a ganglionopathy is associated.

F. **HIV infection**: Distal symmetric polyneuropathy is associated with autonomic manifestations like orthostatic intolerance and gastrointestinal, genitourinary, and sudomotor dysfunction. Cardiovascular autonomic tests may show subclinical sympathetic and parasympathetic dysfunction.

G. **Alcoholic neuropathy**: Patients may present a slowly progressive, predominantly sensory polyneuropathy with pain or burning paresthesia. Autonomic manifestations are limited: erectile dysfunction, palmoplantar hyperhidrosis, and subclinical cardiovagal denervation have been reported.

2. **Which investigations were useful to distinguish among possible diagnoses?**
Blood tests: complete cell count, thyroid function, creatinine, liver function, vitamin B12 and folate levels, protein electrophoresis with immunofixation electrophoresis, rheumatoid factor, ANA, anti-SSA and anti-SSB antibodies, paraneoplastic antibody panel, and HIV testing were normal. CT of the chest/abdomen/pelvis was normal.

3. **What was the most likely diagnosis?**
Diabetic autonomic and somatic length-dependent peripheral polyneuropathy.

4. **How was the patient treated?**
Orthostatic hypotension was treated with nonpharmacological measures and midodrine (see Tables 4.1 and 4.2). Constipation was treated with mild laxatives (Table 4.3).

8.3   Discussion

In our patient, long history of poor blood glucose control and the presence of both sensory and autonomic symptoms narrowed the diagnosis. Causes of chronic polyneuropathy with autonomic manifestations like amyloidosis, metabolic, paraneoplastic, HIV, and alcoholic were ruled out. Damage to nerve fibers due to prolonged exposure to high blood glucose caused a generalized autonomic dysfunction. In our patient, noninvasive autonomic tests were useful to confirm a widespread cardiovagal, cardiovascular sympathetic, and sudomotor denervation.

8.4 Relevant Aspect of Autonomic Dysfunction in Diabetic Neuropathies

Etiology: Factors leading to autonomic nerve damage in diabetes mellitus are multiple including long-standing hyperglycemia, hyperlipidemia, hypertension, obesity, exposure to toxins like ethanol, and possibly genetics. There are loss of distal axonal nerve fibers to peripheral blood vessels and skin, sympathetic ganglia axonal changes, vagal nerve fiber loss, and morphological changes in enteric neurons.

8.5 Clinical Manifestations

Cardiovascular autonomic neuropathy (CAN): The presence of CAN is related with several factors including duration of diabetes, age of the patient, existence of peripheral neuropathy, and glycemic control. The manifestations of CAN are progressive and in early stage may be only subclinical abnormalities of cardiovagal autonomic tests: deep breathing, Valsalva ratio, and HR variability. Later on there are clinical features like resting tachycardia due to cardiovagal denervation, fixed tachycardia caused by both sympathetic and cardiovagal denervation, exercise intolerance, and symptomatic orthostatic hypotension due to a severe sympathetic efferent fiber denervation. Several conditions that contribute to mortality in diabetic patients are associated with CAN: silent myocardial ischemia, cardiovascular instability during surgery procedures, and increased risk for lethal cardiac arrhythmias.

Genitourinary dysfunction: Symptoms of bladder dysfunction due to diabetic autonomic neuropathy occur in the context of a generalized autonomic dysfunction. There is a slowly progressive loss of bladder sensation followed by incomplete bladder emptying that can lead finally to urinary retention with overflow incontinence. In men a prostatic hypertrophy and in women a gynecological pathology must be excluded. Urodynamic study shows impaired detrusor contractility, reduction in urinary flow, and increased post-micturition residual urine volume. There is compromise of both sensory afferent fibers (decreased micturition sensation) and para-sympathetic efferent fibers to the detrusor muscle. Measurement of increased urine post-residual volume by ultrasonography is useful. In men occur erectile dysfunction and retrograde ejaculation, due to sympathetic denervation.

Gastrointestinal dysfunction: It occurs in diabetic patients with long-standing evolution and peripheral neuropathy. Esophageal complications like gastroesophageal reflux and subclinical esophageal dysmotility may be found; dysphagia is uncommon. Gastroparesis is a common complication; patients present nausea, postprandial vomiting, abdominal distention and pain, bloating, and early satiety. Delayed gastric emptying is shown by a scintigraphy. It may contribute to poor glycemic control, with frequent hypo- and hyperglycemic episodes due to a mismatch between insulin action and carbohydrate absorption. In addition, during episodes of acute hyperglycemia, gastrointestinal motility is reduced. Enteropathy may cause constipation which is common; chronic severe constipation may produce megacolon. Episodes of alternating constipation and profuse nocturnal diarrhea associated with fecal incontinence may be troublesome. Causes other than autonomic dysfunction must be considered for gastrointestinal symptoms.

Sudomotor dysfunction: In length-dependent diabetic polyneuropathy, the patient presents a slowly progressive sweating loss; a distal symmetric anhidrosis in lower limbs is followed by upper limb and lower anterior abdomen anhidrosis and finally by a global anhidrosis. Asymmetrical sweating is found in mononeuropathy and diabetic radiculopathy. Compensatory hyperhidrosis in areas with preserved sweating and gustatory sweating over the face, head, neck, and shoulder can occur. Areas of anhidrosis revealed by thermo-regulatory sweating test show a postganglionic sudomotor dysfunction with local iontophoresis of acetylcholine.

Diagnosis: Motor and sensory nerve conduction studies, noninvasive cardiovascular autonomic tests, and the study of the sudomotor dysfunction pattern allow identifying the distribution and severity of the neuropathy. Distal leg skin biopsy helps to quantify intraepidermal unmyelinated C and thinly myelinated Aδ fiber loss and sweat gland denervation.

In addition to the distal sensorimotor peripheral neuropathy, other forms of diabetic neuropathy may be associated with autonomic manifestations. Distal small painful neuropathy manifests with sudomotor and vasomotor abnormalities in the distal portions of the leg and feet, with no other autonomic involvement. Hypoglycemic neuropathy is a painful neuropathy triggered by rapid fall of blood glucose and may be associated with reduced density of epidermal nerve fibers and manifestation of autonomic failure. This condition, in general, is slowly reversible.

Treatment and prognosis: Adequate control of glycemic level may help to prevent the progression of the neuropathy. Early assessment of subclinical CAN is relevant to advise about perioperative cardiovascular risks. Diabetic patients with autonomic neuropathy show increased morbidity and mortality. CAN is an independent risk factor for overall mortality.

8.6 Key Points

Diabetic autonomic neuropathy is often associated with a sensorimotor polyneuropathy.

Diabetic autonomic dysfunction is a slowly progressive condition, from initial subclinical findings to disabling symptoms like orthostatic hypotension and gastrointestinal dysfunction.

In patients with cardiovascular, urinary, and gastrointestinal symptoms, causes other than autonomic dysfunction must be excluded.

Identification of diabetic patients with CAN is important, for management of a suitable hemodynamic stability during perioperative setting.

Diabetic patients with autonomic neuropathy show increased morbidity, high risk of mortality, and sudden death.

Abstract   Clinical case. Differential diagnosis: Amyloidosis, Diabetic neuropathy, Amyloidosis, Paraneoplastic autonomic neuropathy, Infections: HIV, Chagas disease, Hereditary sensory and autonomic neuropathy. Diagnosis: presence of different types of peripheral polyneuropathy, specific blood tests. Molecular genetic testing for hereditary Amyloidosis. Tissue biopsy. Main autonomic manifestations of Amyloidotic neuropathy: orthostatic hypotension, gastrointestinal, genito-urinary and sudomotor dysfunction. Therapy: Tafamidis and liver transplantation for hereditary type. Prognosis of AL and hereditary Amyloidosis.

8.7   Case 2. Amyloidosis

A 50-year-old man is referred for progressive weakness in the hands and feet as well as cramps and paresthesia in the lower limbs over the past 2 years. He also noted erectile dysfunction, difficulty initiating urination, and orthostatic intolerance, with several syncopal episodes. He had several episodes of abdominal pain and diarrhea, anorexia, and 44-pound weight loss. Over the past 6 months, he had experienced shortness of breath and leg swelling. He was admitted to the emergency department due to syncope. He denies consumption of alcohol, use of illicit drugs, or exposure to toxins. He has no family history of neuropathy. A neurological examination showed normal mental status. Cranial nerve examination was normal, including ocular movements and pupillary reflexes. Motor examination showed weakness and wasting in intrinsic muscles of the feet and hands. Reflexes were absent. Sensory testing showed loss of sensation for pinprick, temperature, light touch, and vibration in stocking and glove distribution.

Autonomic testing showed a severe orthostatic hypotension (OH). Supine blood pressure (BP) was 130/60 mmHg, with a heart rate (HR) of 82 bpm. Standing BP was 68/35 mmHg, with a HR of 82 beats per minute. Beat-to-beat BP responses during the Valsalva maneuver showed absent recovery during late phase II and absent late BP overshoot in phase IV. Cardiovagal tests showed markedly reduced HR responses during deep breathing and reduced Valsalva ratio. Sudomotor tests showed absent sympathetic skin responses in the soles. Nerve conduction studies showed absent motor and sensory action potentials in the median, ulnar, peroneal, and sural nerves. Electromyography showed neurogenic changes in hand and lower limb muscles, consistent with a distal symmetrical axonal polyneuropathy.

8.8   Questions for Consideration

1. **What is the differential diagnosis suggested by clinical evaluation and autonomic testing?**

    A. **Amyloidosis:** Both sporadic light-chain (AL) amyloidosis and transthyretin mutation familial amyloidosis (TTR-FA) may present a pattern of generalized autonomic dysfunction, associated with a distal sensorimotor polyneuropathy.
    B. **Diabetic neuropathy**. Among the different presentations, there is a slowly progressive generalized sensorimotor polyneuropathy associated with a widespread autonomic dysfunction.
    C. **Paraneoplastic autonomic neuropathy**: Most cases present with generalized autonomic dysfunction, including orthostatic hypotension, gastrointestinal symptoms, urinary retention, erectile dysfunction, and sicca syndrome. Association with a peripheral neuropathy or with central nervous system disorder is frequent.

D. **Infections:** Autonomic dysfunction may occur in HIV; HIV-seropositive patients with advanced disease may present a generalized autonomic failure. In leprosy neuropathy, there is a focal small fiber compromise of sensory, vasomotor, and sudomotor fibers; a widespread autonomic dysfunction is rare. In chronic stage of Chagas disease, there are gastrointestinal symptoms due to megaesophagus and megacolon; cardiovascular sympathetic and parasympathetic dysfunction can also occur.

E. **Hereditary sensory and autonomic neuropathy (HSAN).** The type I HSAN may present in adult life with neuropathic pain and progressive distal sensory loss; the main autonomic manifestation is distal anhidrosis or hyperhidrosis.

2. **Which investigations were useful to distinguish among possible diagnoses?**
   Blood glucose, paraneoplastic antibody panel, and HIV testing were normal. Immunoelectrophoresis showed an elevated monoclonal immunoglobulin L-chain peak. Two-dimensional CT of the chest/abdomen/pelvis was normal. Abdominal fat aspirate using Congo red staining showed amyloid deposits. Echocardiography (2-D echo) showed increased ventricular wall and septal thickness, with granular "sparkling" image. Molecular genetic testing excluded TTR-FA.

3. **What was the most likely diagnosis?**
   Sporadic AL amyloidosis.

4. **How was the patient treated?**
   Orthostatic hypotension was treated with general measures and midodrine (see Tables 4.1 and 4.2), for amyloidosis. Amyloidosis was treated with a combination of melphalan and prednisone.

8.9   Discussion

In this patient, alternative causes of chronic autonomic dysfunction with peripheral polyneuropathy, such as diabetes mellitus, paraneoplastic, infections, and hereditary neuropathy, were excluded. The presence of systemic manifestations, including severe weight loss, diarrhea, dyspnea, and leg swelling, led to consider an amyloidotic neuropathy. Our patient had the most frequent pattern of AL amyloidotic neuropathy, which is a classic example of polyneuropathy associated with generalized autonomic failure. Isolated autonomic dysfunction is a less frequent pattern. Our patient showed normal pupils. However, Argyll Robertson pupil and scalloped pupil due to local amyloid deposits in ciliary nerves can also be found. Other hereditary amyloidoses, including gelsolin amyloidosis, show only minor or no autonomic manifestations.

8.10   Relevant Aspect of Autonomic Dysfunction in Amyloidotic Neuropathies

Etiology. The amyloidoses are a group of diseases that have in common the extracellular deposition of pathologic, insoluble fibrils in various tissues and organs. In AL amyloidosis, plasma cells produce excessive monoclonal light-chain proteins. In autosomal dominant TTR-FA, the liver produces a high amount of TTR, which is a small transport protein for thyroxine and retinol. There are about 126 different genetic variations in TTR-FA. Among others, in non-TTR-FA, there are mutations of apolipoprotein A-1 and A-2, gelsolin actin-binding plasma protein, fibrinogen A alpha-chain, lysozyme, and cystatin C.

8.11   Clinical Manifestations

Cardiovascular dysfunction: Symptomatic OH is frequent in both AL amyloidosis and TTR-FA; subclinical OH may also occur in some cases. Amyloid deposits in both sympathetic ganglia and efferent sympathetic fibers may contribute to vasomotor dysfunction. Orthostatic hypotension may be an initial manifestation in AL-type amyloidosis and early-onset TTR-FA. A cardiac conduction disorder may be secondary to amyloid infiltration or autonomic dysfunction.

Gastrointestinal dysfunction: In both AL amyloidosis and TTR-FA, several factors contribute to gastroparesis, constipation, and diarrhea. These include amyloid infiltration of the smooth muscle, autonomic dysfunction, intestinal inflammation, and bacterial overgrowth. Gastric retention is common in hereditary TTR-FA. Intestinal pseudo-obstruction can occur. Amyloid deposits may affect the vagus nerve fibers, celiac ganglion, and enteric neurons.

Genitourinary: Urinary symptoms, including dysuria and urinary retention, typically occur later in the evolution of amyloid autonomic neuropathy. The main urodynamic findings are impaired bladder sensation and underactive detrusor muscle resulting in inability to void and excessive post-void residual urine. Detrusor underactivity may reflect postganglionic cholinergic nerve fiber denervation. In men, erectile dysfunction is an early feature that might precede sensory symptoms of neuropathy.

Sudomotor: The most frequent finding is a length-dependent symmetrical distal anhidrosis; a generalized or a patchy distribution of anhidrosis is less frequent. This reflects an early damage of small sympathetic sudomotor fibers.

Diagnosis: Serum and urine immunoelectrophoresis to measure light-chain protein is the main initial laboratory test to detect AL amyloidosis. Bone marrow biopsy is used to detect plasma cell dyscrasia. Subcutaneous abdominal fat aspiration has a sensitivity of 80% in detecting systemic amyloidosis. In both AL amyloidosis and familial amyloidosis, immunohistochemical study and mass spectrometry amyloid typing are useful tools to identify different amyloid proteins. Molecular genetic testing using targeted mutation analysis and sequence analysis methods are used for diagnosis of familial amyloidosis.

Treatment and prognosis: The main treatment for familial amyloidosis is liver transplantation. Tafamidis, a drug that can stabilize TTR protein, may be useful at early stages of the disease. Patients with AL-type amyloidosis should be considered for stem cell transplantation. If not eligible, treatment with alkylating agents, corticosteroids, immunomodulatory drugs, and proteasome inhibitors should be considered. Immunosuppressive treatment may improve survival, mainly when the therapy provoked a reduction in monoclonal protein. The median survival of patients with AL amyloidotic neuropathy is in the range of 13–35 months; survival in AL has improved over the last decades. In TTR-FA, survival is up to 15 years and has improved with liver transplantation.

8.12 Key Points

- Both sporadic AL amyloidosis and TTR-FA subtypes show important autonomic dysfunction; other rare familial subtypes may show only minor autonomic symptoms.
- Autonomic dysfunction commonly reflects amyloid deposition in autonomic nerves, peripheral organs, or both
- Autonomic symptoms may precede other neuropathic or systemic manifestations, so the diagnosis of amyloidosis may be delayed.
- In amyloid neuropathy, autonomic testing may yield abnormal results before clinical autonomic manifestations occur.
- In amyloid neuropathy, OH and diarrhea are disabling manifestations.
- Early detection of amyloidosis allows early treatment, improving the management of different organs' failure and survival.

Bibliography

1. Fealey RD, Low PA, Thomas JE. Thermoregulatory sweating abnormalities in diabetes mellitus. Mayo Clin Proc. 1989;64(6):617–28.
2. Low PA, Benrud-Larson LM, Sletten DM, Opfer-Gehrking TL, Weigand SD, O'Brien PC, Suarez GA, Dyck PJ. Autonomic symptoms and diabetic neuropathy: a population-based study. Diabetes Care. 2004;27:2942–7.
3. Vinik AI, Ziegler D. Diabetic cardiovascular autonomic neuropathy. Circulation. 2007;115:387–97.
4. Freeman R. Diabetic autonomic neuropathy. Handb Clin Neurol. 2014;126:63–79.
5. Liu Y, Billiet J, Ebenezer GJ, Ebenezer GJ, Pan B, Hauer P, Wei J, Polydefkis M. Factors influencing sweat gland innervation in diabetes. Neurology. 2015;84:1652–9.
6. Wang AK, Fealey RD, Gehrking TL, Low PA. Patterns of neuropathy and autonomic failure in patients with amyloidosis. Mayo Clin Proc. 2008;83:1226–30.
7. Kim DH, Zeldenrust SR, Low PA, Dyck PJ. Quantitative sensation and autonomic test abnormalities in transthyretin amyloidosis polyneuropathy. Muscle Nerve. 2009;40:363–70.
8. Plante-Bordeneuve V, Said G. Familial amyloid polyneuropathy. Lancet Neurol. 2011;10:1086–97.
9. Chao CC, Huang CM, Chiang HH, Luo KR, Kan HW, Yang NC, et al. Sudomotor innervation in transthyretin amyloid neuropathy: pathology and functional correlates. Ann Neurol. 2015;78(2):272–83.
10. Gertz MA. Immunoglobulin light chain amyloidosis: 2016 update on diagnosis, prognosis, and treatment. Am J Hematol. 2016;91:947–56.

Chapter 9
Autonomic Failure in Subacute Sensory Ganglioneuronopathies

Juan Idiaquez, Eduardo Benarroch, and Martin Nogues

9.1   Case 9. Sjögren Syndrome

A 43-year-old woman presented for evaluation of excessive sweating on the left trunk over the past 4 years. She also complained of mild paresthesia in the left foot that progressed to involve both feet. After several months she noticed instability during walking. More recently, she started developing numbness in the right side of the face and moderate symptoms of orthostatic intolerance, including dizziness and light-headedness on standing. She has also noticed constipation

J. Idiaquez (✉)
Universidad de Valparaiso, Viña del Mar, Chile
e-mail: idiaquez@123.cl

E. Benarroch
Mayo Clinic, Rochester, MN, USA
e-mail: benarroch@mayo.edu

M. Nogues
Clinica Fleni, Buenos Aires, Argentina
e-mail: mnogues@fleni.org.ar

© Springer International Publishing AG 2018   87
J. Idiaquez et al. (eds.), *Evaluation and Management of Autonomic Disorders*,
https://doi.org/10.1007/978-3-319-72251-1_9

and dry eyes and mouth. General examination was normal. Neurological examination showed mild sensory ataxia. Mental status examination was normal. Cranial nerve examination showed lack of pupil reaction to light and tonic response to convergence, without ptosis and oculomotor abnormalities. There was also lack of pinprick sensation in the face. Muscle strength was normal but deep tendon reflexes were absent. Sensory examination showed reduced proprioception in toes. On autonomic testing, supine blood pressure was 111/68 mmHg with a heart rate of 82 bpm; standing blood pressure was 90/54 mmHg with a heart rate of 96 bpm. There were reduced heart rate response to deep breathing and reduced Valsalva ratio, indicating cardiovagal denervation. Pupils constricted upon local application of diluted pilocarpine (0.00625%) indicating parasympathetic denervation of pupils with denervation supersensitivity. Thermoregulatory sweating test (iodine-starch) showed an area of segmental anhidrosis in the right trunk.

9.2   Questions for Consideration

1. **What was the differential diagnosis suggested by clinical evaluation and autonomic testing?**
   The presence of autonomic dysfunction with sensory neuropathy suggests the following possible diagnoses:

   A. Paraneoplastic Autonomic Ganglionopathy
      This disorder presents with subacute widespread sympathetic and parasympathetic dysfunction, including orthostatic hypotension with disabling orthostatic intolerance and syncope, severe gastrointestinal symptoms mainly constipation, urinary retention, dry eyes and mouth, and difficulty in vision in bright light due to pupillary dysfunction. Our patient presented with longstanding moderate autonomic manifestations with segmental anhidrosis and compensatory hyperhidrosis, orthostatic intolerance, and constipation. Our patient did not present urinary dysfunction. Many patients

with paraneoplastic autonomic dysfunction present a concomitant peripheral polyneuropathy or ganglionopathy or central nervous system dysfunction. Paraneoplastic neuropathy presents subacute onset, while our patient's symptoms showed a slow progression.

B. Systemic Lupus Erythematosus (SLE)

Patients may present with sensory or sensorimotor neuropathy, but symptoms of autonomic dysfunction are not common; LES patients may present only subclinical autonomic abnormalities like cardiovagal and sudomotor dysfunction. Our patient presented with sudomotor symptoms, orthostatic intolerance, and constipation associated with sensory symptoms.

Sjögren Syndrome.

2. **Which investigations were useful to distinguish among possible diagnoses?**

Nerve conduction studies showed normal motor conductions, with reduced sensory nerve action potential amplitude in the median and sural nerves. Antibody testing showed positive SSA (anti-Ro) and SSB (anti-La) antibodies and elevated d rheumatoid factor. Antinuclear antibodies (ANA), antibodies to double-strand DNA, ANA subtypes such as Sm, and ribonucleoprotein (RNP) showed low titers; complement was normal. Paraneoplastic antibodies, including antineuronal nuclear antibody type 1 (ANNA-1, anti-Hu) and ANNA-2 (anti-Ri), Purkinje cell cytoplasmic antibody type 2 (PCA-2), amphiphysin antibody, and collapsin response mediator protein 5 (CRMP-5) were all negative. Schirmer's test showed reduced basal tear secretion. Minor salivary gland biopsy (lip) showed chronic lymphocytic sialoadenitis. Cervical cord MRI showed increased T2 signal in the posterior columns.

3. **What was the most likely diagnosis**?

Clinical signs and electrophysiological signs of sensory ganglionopathy associated with a long-standing autonomic dysfunction, with high titers of SSA and SSB, and with salivary gland chronic inflammation support the diagnosis of Sjögren syndrome (SS).

4. **How was the patient treated?**

Orthostatic hypotension was treated (see Tables 4.1 and 4.2) with a combination of fludrocortisone and midodrine. The patient also received immunotherapy for her extraglandular manifestations (autonomic and sensory neuropathy).

9.3   Discussion

The present case showed autonomic dysfunction and sensory ganglionopathy. Paraneoplastic autonomic ganglionopathy and SLE neuropathy were excluded by the elevated titers of SSA and SSB and the negative titers of paraneoplastic antibodies and the low titers of antibodies in the SLE panel. In our patient, main autonomic manifestation was segmental anhidrosis in the trunk with compensatory hyperhidrosis, which is not the pattern of sudomotor dysfunction in paraneoplastic neuropathy. Also the patient showed moderate orthostatic intolerance and constipation without urinary dysfunction, while in paraneoplastic condition, there is a severe generalized autonomic dysfunction. In addition the slow progression of autonomic symptoms differs with subacute presentation of paraneoplastic autonomic complaints.

9.4   Relevant Aspect of Autonomic Dysfunction in Sjögren Syndrome

Etiology: Sjögren syndrome is a systemic autoimmune disease that primarily affects the exocrine glands (mainly the salivary and lacrimal glands). Most of SS patients present with sicca syndrome (dry eyes and dry mouth) and parotid gland enlargement, but in about 30% of SS patients, there are rheumatologic, neurologic, pulmonary, or gastrointestinal manifestations. The clinical presentation of autonomic dysfunction in SS varies from mild symptoms to a more severe autonomic failure. SS is often detected several years after the occurrence of autonomic manifestations.

9.5   Clinical Manifestations

Orthostatic Hypotension

Orthostatic intolerance is a common symptom among patients with SS, but the occurrence of severe symptomatic OH is less frequent. Disabling OH occurs in cases with generalized autonomic failure. Autonomic test may show abnormal blood pressure profile (reduced late phase II and IV) during the Valsalva maneuver. Low supine plasma levels of norepinephrine without increase on standing and reduced cardiac MIBG uptake reflect peripheral sympathetic denervation. In the majority of SS cases, the presence of OH occurs in combination with sensory ganglionopathy, but some patients may present with a predominantly generalized autonomic failure. SS patients with orthostatic intolerance may show postural tachycardia without OH, which may be related to a moderate sympathetic dysfunction or to a neurogenic postural orthostatic tachycardia syndrome (POTS). Morphological studies in SS show loss of sensory and autonomic ganglion neurons, with infiltration of CD8+ T cells.

9.6   Sweating Dysfunction

Sweating symptoms are present in SS patients with sensory ganglionopathy, but they can occur in isolation or in combination with Adie pupils. Patients may present areas of segmental anhidrosis with compensatory hyperhidrosis, in areas of preserved sweating. Morphological studies show that sympathetic ganglion neuron loss may present a variable segmental distribution, which is in keeping with the segmental distribution of anhidrosis.

9.7   Pupillary Symptoms

Patients may present bilateral Adie pupils, with mydriasis nonreactive to light and tonic constrictor response. Less frequent finding is unilateral Adie pupil, presenting with anisocoria. Tonic pupils are present in patients with sensory ganglionopathy but can occur as an early manifestation of SS. They may also reflect degeneration of ciliary ganglion, receptor blockade by autoantibodies against M3-muscarinic acetylcholine receptors, or both. Pharmacological test had shown parasympathetic pupillary denervation in SS.

9.8   Gastrointestinal and Urinary Symptoms

Chronic gastrointestinal symptoms including abdominal pain, constipation, and diarrhea are reported in SS cases with generalized autonomic failure. Functional studies had shown gastrointestinal dysmotility and slow colonic transit, with normal rectal sphincter EMG. Urinary dysfunction is mild and less frequent and can occur in the context of generalized autonomic failure. Urodynamic studies show normal bladder capacity and without detrusor overactivity or low compliance. Autoantibodies against M3-muscarinic acetylcholine receptors may account for gastrointestinal dysmotility and bladder dysfunction.

9.9   Diagnosis

The diagnostic criteria of SS include the detection of autoantibodies (ANA, RF, SSA, and SSB) in serum and histological analysis of biopsied salivary gland tissue (showing lymphocytic infiltration of the affected tissue or the deposition of the immune complex). Schirmer's test confirms reduced tear secretion, as does slit-lamp exam with vital dye staining. Salivary flow rate, and/or nuclear scintigraphy evaluation of the salivary glandular function. Ganglionic acetylcholine receptor antibody titers in plasma may be elevated in patients with symptomatic autonomic failure.

9.10   Treatment and Prognosis

There are small series that show good therapeutic response of orthostatic intolerance and gastrointestinal symptoms with intravenous immunoglobulin and rituximab. In some patients with SS and autonomic failure with elevated titer of ganglionic AChR antibody, autonomic symptoms may improve with immunotherapy.

9.11   Key Points

- Autonomic dysfunction may be an early manifestation of SS and can precede the diagnosis of disease for several years.
- Clinical autonomic involvement in SS tends to be chronic and ranges from modest focal disorders (pupillary dysfunction, segmental anhidrosis) to a disabling generalized autonomic failure.
- Autonomic symptoms in SS often occur in association with signs of sensory ganglionopathy (ataxic and/or painful type), but there are some cases with predominantly generalized autonomic failure.
- Autonomic symptoms and signs in SS patients may improve with immunotherapy, in particular in those patients with elevated titer of ganglionic acetylcholine receptor antibody.

Bibliography

1. Newton JL, Frith J, Powell D, Hackett K, Wilton K, Bowman S, et al. Autonomic symptoms are common and are associated with overall symptom burden and disease activity in primary Sjogren's syndrome. Ann Rheum Dis. 2012;71:1973–9.

2. Mukaino A, Nakane S, Higuchi O, Nakamura H, Miyagi T, Shiroma K, et al. Insights from the ganglionic acetylcholine receptor autoantibodies in patients with Sjögren's syndrome. Mod Rheumatol. 2016;26(5):708–15.
3. Mori K, Iijima M, Koike H, Hattori N, Tanaka F, Watanabe H, et al. The wide spectrum of clinical manifestations in Sjögren's syndrome-associated neuropathy. Brain. 2005;128:2518–34.
4. Sakakibara R, Hirano S, Asahina M, Sawai S, Nemoto Y, Hiraga A, et al. Primary Sjogren's syndrome presenting with generalized autonomic failure. Eur J Neurol. 2004;11:635–8.
5. Goodman BP, Crepeau A, Dhawan PS, Khoury JA, Harris LA. Spectrum of autonomic nervous system impairment in Sjögren syndrome. Neurologist. 2017;22:127–30.
6. Goodman BP. Immunoresponsive autonomic neuropathy in Sjögren syndrome-case series and literature review. Am J Ther. 2017. https://doi.org/10.1097/MJT.0000000000000583.

Chapter 10
Autonomic Failure and Acute Motor Weakness

Juan Idiaquez, Eduardo Benarroch, and Martin Nogues

10.1 Case 1. Guillain-Barré Syndrome

A 29-year-old man presented for evaluation of progressive symmetrical ascending muscle weakness affecting first the lower and then the upper limbs over the past 2 days. He was admitted to the hospital. Neurological examination showed normal mental status. Cranial nerve examinations showed bilateral facial nerve palsy. Motor examination showed flaccid tetraplegia with absence of deep tendon reflexes. Sensory examination was normal. Over the following 3 days, he

J. Idiaquez (✉)
Universidad de Valparaiso, Viña del Mar, Chile
e-mail: idiaquez@123.cl

E. Benarroch
Mayo Clinic, Rochester, MN, USA
e-mail: benarroch@mayo.edu

M. Nogues
Clinica Fleni, Buenos Aires, Argentina
e-mail: mnogues@fleni.org.ar

© Springer International Publishing AG 2018   95
J. Idiaquez et al. (eds.), *Evaluation and Management of Autonomic Disorders*,
https://doi.org/10.1007/978-3-319-72251-1_10

developed weakness of neck and trunk muscles and tachypnea. He was admitted to the intensive care unit for mechanical ventilation. Cardiovascular monitoring showed blood pressure (BP) fluctuations, with two episodes of severe hypertension with elevated plasma norepinephrine. He also experienced episodes of sinus tachycardia or bradycardia, occasionally provoked by tracheal suction or painful stimuli. The patient had urinary retention and abdominal pain with constipation (X-ray image showed ileus) that lasted several days.

10.2   Questions for Consideration

1. **What was the differential diagnosis suggested by clinical evaluation and autonomic testing?**
   The presence of autonomic dysfunction with subacute symmetrical motor polyneuropathy suggests the following diagnoses:

   A. Guillain-Barré Syndrome (GBS)
      GBS may be preceded by a viral infection or vaccination that induced an autoimmune response targeting roots and peripheral nerves. Typically there is an acute progression of symmetric limb weakness and areflexia. Autonomic manifestations may occur early and mainly in cases with severe motor deficits and ventilatory failure. Sympathetic and parasympathetic cardiovascular dysfunction manifested by BP and heart rate (HR) instability. Transient urinary retention, constipation, and sudomotor dysfunction may be present.
   B. Botulism
      The neurotoxin (produced by Clostridium botulinum) blocks presynaptic cholinergic transmission, causing muscle weakness and autonomic dysfunction. Patient history includes ingestion of poorly preserved food, iatrogenic overdose in therapeutic use of the toxin, or wounds. Motor deficit in botulism, unlike typical GNS, is characterized by descending pattern of weakness

and preserved deep tendon reflexes. Autonomic dysfunction in botulism reflects impaired cholinergic transmission and includes bilateral dilated and unreactive pupils, dry mouth, urinary retention, and constipation.

C. Porphyria

Porphyria is a rare hereditary disorder of heme (part of the hemoglobin molecule) metabolism; there is increased accumulation and elimination of porphyrins and their precursors. Acute intermittent porphyria (AIP), variegate porphyria, and hereditary coproporphyria may present with neurological compromise. In AIP, patients suffer from episodes of severe abdominal pain followed by motor axonal polyneuropathy and autonomic dysfunction: tachycardia, constipation, and hypertension.

D. Lambert-Eaton Syndrome (LEMS)

LEMS is an autoimmune disorder of neuromuscular transmission, caused by antibodies directed against presynaptic P/Q-type voltage-gated calcium channels. In about 50% of cases, there is an association with small cell lung cancer. In LEMS patients, the occurrence of myasthenic symptoms may be associated with an acute cholinergic dysfunction including dry mouth, hypohidrosis, and orthostatic hypotension.

2. **Which investigations were useful to distinguish among possible diagnoses?**

Blood tests: complete blood cell count, electrolytes, hemoglobin A1c, HIV testing, anti-hepatitis C, and antinuclear antibodies were all normal. Porphyrin levels in blood, urine, and stool were normal. Nerve conduction and EMG study were compatible with a demyelinating polyneuropathy. High-frequency repetitive nerve stimulation was normal. Cerebrospinal fluid showed elevated protein concentration with a normal cell count.

3. **What was the most likely diagnosis?**

GBS.

4. **How was the patient treated?**
   The patient was treated with IV immunoglobulin. Intensive
   unit care management included mechanical ventilation
   and cardiovascular monitoring; episodes of hypertensive
   crisis were treated with labetalol IV. Ileus was treated with
   suspension of enteral feed and parenteral nutrition. A ster-
   ile closed urinary drainage system was used during the
   urine retention episode.

10.3   Discussion

Our patient presented severe blood pressure fluctuations,
with sympathetic hyperactivity which is not observed in botulism. In GBS occurs an ascending symmetrical motor weakness with absent reflexes, while botulism shows a descending
pattern of motor deficits with preserved reflexes. In AIP
severe abdominal pain and psychiatric symptoms are associated with motor axonal polyneuropathy. Autonomic dysfunction in AIP can present with sympathetic hyperactivity with
tachycardia and hypertension. In LEMS there is cholinergic
dysfunction but no BP fluctuations present. Different mechanisms may be responsible for autonomic dysfunction in GBS:
nerve fiber injury caused by neurotoxic cytokines, lymphocytic infiltration, or circulating autoantibodies. Antibodies
again to ganglionic acetylcholine receptor may contribute to
autonomic dysfunction in GBS. Baroreflex impairment due
to demyelination of baroreceptor afferents is likely the cause
of BP and HR fluctuations.

10.4   Relevant Aspect of Autonomic
Dysfunction in GBS Syndrome

Clinical Manifestations

Cardiovascular Autonomic Dysfunction

Blood pressure instability: Episodes of hypotension and
hypertension and sympathetic hyperactivity with paroxysmal

or persistent hypertension may be a life-threatening complication. There is an association between BP increase and severity of the disease. Mechanisms involved in sympathetic instability are baroreceptor afferent denervation and elevated plasma levels of epinephrine and norepinephrine due to a failure of catecholamine uptake and denervation hypersensitivity. Blood pressure fluctuation and hypertensive crises may elicit posterior reversible encephalopathy syndrome; baroreflex impairment may contribute to the syndrome of inappropriate secretion of antidiuretic hormone. Management of BP fluctuation requires permanent monitoring and avoiding precipitating factors, particularly pain and visceral distension. OH may be an initial manifestation and may occur during the evolution when the patient is in a sitting or standing position.

Heart rate: Transient sinus tachycardia is frequent but sustained tachycardia and other severe tachyarrhythmias such as atrial and ventricular arrhythmias are less frequent. Bradycardia due to cardiovagal hyperactivity may lead to heart block and asystole, which can be life-threatening. Severe bradycardia may be caused by tracheal suctioning or by drug therapy. Patients with severe motor and ventilatory dysfunction have more risk to develop BP fluctuations and bradycardia. Sustained cardiovascular abnormalities in GBS may be secondary to sepsis, lung embolism, severe pain, dehydration, and myocardial damage.

Myocardial compromise: Takotsubo cardiomyopathy is a transient left ventricular apical ballooning cardiomyopathy, possibly related with sympathetic hyperactivity and elevation of plasma catecholamine levels. A direct effect of catecholamines may elicit contraction band necrosis of cardiac myocytes. The ECG shows ST-segment elevation and T-wave inversion. There is an increase in creatine kinase-MB and cardiac troponin concentrations. Echocardiography shows left ventricular apical akinesis and ballooning with basal hyperkinesis. Takotsubo cardiomyopathy is often benign but in some cases can be associated with neurogenic pulmonary edema, provoked cardiogenic shock, and cardiac arrest.

Gastrointestinal: Adynamic ileus occurs in about 15% of severe GBS patients and may be a presenting feature of the disease. Upper ileus may present with pain and abdominal distention, lower ileus with alternating diarrhea and constipation. Adynamic ileus during early stage of the disease is associated with a widespread autonomic dysfunction, while ileus occurring during the recovery phase may be associated to immobility. Serial abdominal X-ray is useful for early detection. Possibly gut denervation is responsible for ileus.

Genitourinary: Urinary symptoms occur in about 25% of patients and are less common than cardiovascular symptoms. Urinary retention secondary to detrusor underactivity is transient in classic GBS. In axonal variant of GBS, urinary dysfunction may persist.

Sudomotor: Episodes of generalized hyperhidrosis can infrequently occur. There are reports of patchy areas of anhidrosis with the thermoregulatory sweat test and denervation of sudomotor fibers in skin biopsy.

10.5   Diagnosis: Treatment and Prognosis

Early monitoring of ventilatory capacity and cardiovascular function is crucial. Hypotensive episodes could be treated with IV fluid for volume expansion and elevation of the legs. Hypertension requires careful management. Transient and moderate episodes of increased BP must be observed, and only severe hypertension associated with potential cardiac ischemia or brain hemorrhage risk must be treated. Hypotensive drugs may cause severe hypotension due to baroreflex failure and denervation hypersensitivity. Heart block and asystole may require temporary or permanent pacemaker placement. Motor weakness and autonomic dysfunction improve with IV immunoglobulin or with plasmapheresis in the majority of patients. Hypotensive drugs with short half-life are useful. Mortality rate varies between 3 and 7%, patients die during the acute period, and causes are ventilatory insufficiency, pulmonary complications, and autonomic dysfunction.

10.6 Key Points

During acute phase of GBS with severe evolution, cardiovascular autonomic dysfunction may be a life-threatening complication. Cardiac and hemodynamic monitoring is essential.

In GBS blood pressure instability may cause severe hypertensive crisis and hypotensive episodes; HR instability may cause transient tachycardia and tachyarrhythmias and episodes of bradycardia leading to asystole and heart block.

Gastrointestinal autonomic dysfunction may manifest with transient adynamic ileus during the acute phase of GBS evolution, in combination with cardiovascular and urinary dysfunction.

In classic GBS transient urinary retention caused by underactivity of detrusor muscle is less frequent than cardiovascular autonomic dysfunction.

In the majority of patients with classic GBS, both motor weakness and autonomic dysfunction improve with IV immunoglobulin or plasmapheresis.

Bibliography

1. Mukerji S, Aloka F, Farooq MU, Kassab MY, Abela GS. Cardiovascular complications of the Guillain-Barré syndrome. Am J Cardiol. 2009;104:1452–5.
2. Sakakibara R, Uchiyama T, Kuwabara S, Mori M, Ito T, Yamamoto T, et al. Prevalence and mechanism of bladder dysfunction in Guillain-Barré syndrome. Neurourol Urodyn. 2009;28:432–7.
3. Van den Berg B, Walgaard C, Drenthen J, Fokke C, Jacobs BC, van Doorn PA. Guillain-Barré syndrome: pathogenesis, diagnosis, treatment and prognosis. Nat Rev Neurol. 2014;10:469–82.
4. Nakane S, Higuchi O, Hamada Y, Maeda Y, Mukaino A, Sakai W, Kusunoki S, Matsuo H. Ganglionic acetylcholine receptor autoantibodies in patients with Guillain-Barré syndrome. J Neuroimmunol. 2016;295-296:54–9.
5. Willison HJ, Jacobs BC, van Doorn PA. Guillain-Barré syndrome. Lancet. 2016;388:717–27.
6. Anandan C, Khuder SA, Koffman BM. Prevalence of autonomic dysfunction in hospitalized patients with Guillain-Barré syndrome. Muscle Nerve. 2017;56:331–3.

Chapter 11
Distal Painful Autonomic Neuropathy

Juan Idiaquez, Eduardo Benarroch, and Martin Nogues

11.1 Case 1. Small Fiber Neuropathy

A 64-year-old man in the last 4 years has noted a history of slowly progressive nocturnal paresthesia with burning, prickling, and pain in both feet. At that time, a primary care consultation showed body mass index of 31 (obese range), glycemia, and hemoglobin A1c were normal. High serum triglyceride levels = 210 mg/dL, and impaired glucose tolerance test was found. He was advised to do a lifestyle modification (diet and exercise). The patient did not follow medical

J. Idiaquez (✉)
Universidad de Valparaiso, Viña del Mar, Chile
e-mail: idiaquez@123.cl

E. Benarroch
Mayo Clinic, Rochester, MN, USA
e-mail: benarroch@mayo.edu

M. Nogues
Clinica Fleni, Buenos Aires, Argentina
e-mail: mnogues@fleni.org.ar

© Springer International Publishing AG 2018   103
J. Idiaquez et al. (eds.), *Evaluation and Management of Autonomic Disorders*,
https://doi.org/10.1007/978-3-319-72251-1_11

indications. He noticed worsening of his painful paresthesia. Also he complained of skin intolerance to socks and bed sheets. A recent medical evaluation showed a fasting blood glucose level of 190 mg/dL and hemoglobin A1c = 7.5. He did not refer alcohol or drug consumption. Neurological evaluation: normal cognitive status. Cranial nerves: normal function. Motor examination: normal muscle strength and reflexes in upper and lower limbs. Sensory test: pinprick and temperature sensory loss, with normal light touch and vibration on feet. Hyperalgesia and allodynia were also found on feet. Autonomic testing showed normal blood pressure and heart rate change on standing. Valsalva: normal phase II and IV. Cardiovagal test (deep breathing): abnormal HR change. Sudomotor: Quantitative sudomotor axon reflex test (QSART) in the ankle showed decreased sweat volume. Nerve conduction: Peroneal motor conduction was normal. Sural and superficial peroneal nerve amplitudes were normal. Punch skin biopsy showed reduced intraepidermal fiber density (IENFD) in the distal leg.

11.2   Questions for Consideration

1. **What are the differential diagnosis suggested by clinical evaluation and autonomic testing?**
   Metabolic/nutritional: Diabetes mellitus and impaired glucose tolerance, rapid glycemic control, thyroid dysfunction, hyperlipidemia, vitamin B12, B1, and B6 deficiency or excess

   Autoimmune: Sjögren syndrome, systemic lupus erythematosus, celiac disease, vasculitis, sarcoidosis

   Paraneoplastic: Lung cancer, multiple myeloma, and monoclonal gammapathies

   Drug toxicity and toxics: Statins, metronidazole, chemotherapeutic agents, alcohol, and heavy metals (thallium, mercury, arsenic)

   Infectious: HIV, hepatitis C, influenza, leprosy, and Lyme

Amyloidosis: Sporadic AL subtype and TTR-FA

Hereditary: Fabry disease, hereditary sensory and autonomic neuropathies (HSAN), sodium channel mutations ($Na_v1.7$, Na_v 1.8, Na_v 1.9), and Tangier disease

2. **Which investigations are useful to distinguish among possible diagnosis?**
   Blood test: Complete cell count, thyroid function, creatinine, liver function, vitamin B12 and folate levels, protein electrophoresis with immunofixation electrophoresis, rheumatoid factor, ANA, anti-SSA and SSB antibodies, tissue transglutaminase IgA antibody, deamidated gliadin IgA and IgG antibodies paraneoplastic antibodies panel, HIV testing, and antibody testing for hepatitis C virus—all were normal. CT chest/abdomen/pelvis was normal.

3. **What was the most likely diagnosis?**
   Length-dependent small fiber neuropathy associated with type 2 diabetes mellitus and hyperlipidemia

4. **How was the patient treated?**
   Neuropathic pain was treated with pregabalin and duloxetine. Blood glucose level was stabilized with diet and metformin. Dyslipidemia was treated with diet.

11.3   Discussion

Our patient presents with symptoms, signs, and sudomotor and skin biopsy tests, compatible with a length-dependent small fiber compromise. There is wide spectrum of disorders associated with this specific neuropathy from metabolic condition like our diabetic patient to rare hereditary diseases. In diabetes mellitus, small fiber denervation may precede the occurrence of large fiber involvement. This patient did not show prominent autonomic symptoms. Subclinical sudomotor and cardiovagal dysfunction were present. Considering that conventional nerve conduction studies are normal, detection of hypohidrosis or anhidrosis in a length-dependent distribution is a useful tool for study of small fiber dysfunction. It is important to consider that in some conditions like Sjögren syndrome, sweating loss may occur in a non-length-dependent distribution in focal areas, such as the face or trunk. Autonomic symptoms like orthostatic intolerance, constipation, micturition, and erectile dysfunction may be present in some patients, and it may precede the manifestation of the associated condition. It may happen in cancer, Sjögren syndrome, amyloidosis, and Fabry disease among others. Thus a follow-up of patients with "idiopathic" small fiber neuropathy is crucial. Recent studies had identified several sodium channel mutation associated with painful small fiber neuropathy, which may present distal or proximal (eyes, jaw) paroxysmal pain crisis.

11.4 Relevant Aspect of Autonomic Dysfunction in Small Fiber Neuropathies

Etiology: A selective damage to small myelinated $A\delta$ and unmyelinated C nerve fibers is found in a wide range of disorders. Mechanisms that cause this denervation depend on each pathological condition.

11.5 Autonomic Manifestations

Sudomotor and vasomotor dysfunction: Patients may present feet changes like excessive coldness and skin atrophy, shiny and dry skin, and occasionally excessive sweating. The presence of distal hypohidrosis or anhidrosis is frequent, and it may be shown by different sudomotor tests. Distal vasomotor dysfunction in lower limbs is frequent; both vasoconstriction and vasodilatation reflex mechanisms of peripheral blood vessels are compromised.

Other autonomic dysfunction: Occasionally orthostatic hypotension is found, and autonomic reflex tests may show cardiovagal denervation. Gastrointestinal and genitourinary symptoms are not disabling.

Diagnosis. The diagnosis is based upon:

1. Intraepidermal fiber density (IENFD) loss by punch skin biopsy.
2. Quantitative sensory is a psychophysical testing that may detect distal sensory loss.
3. Sweating tests: thermoregulatory sweating test may show distal anhidrosis; QSART in distal leg is abnormal in about 80% of patients. Sympathetic skin responses (SSR) and Sudoscan may be useful.
4. Other tests: cardiovascular reflex test dysfunction is less frequent than sudomotor denervation.

Corneal confocal microscopy can detect small fiber corneal denervation. Laser Doppler flowmetry may show abnormal distal vasomotor reflexes. Quantification of sweat gland dermal fiber loss may contribute to diagnosis.

Treatment and prognosis: For management of pain, a multidisciplinary approach is useful. Recognition of a treatable underlying disorder and their specific treatment improve the prognosis.

11.6   Key Points

In small fiber neuropathy, there is a selective compromise of sensory and autonomic fibers in a length-dependent pattern; a non-length-dependent distribution of fiber loss is less frequent.

There is a heterogeneous group of conditions associated with small fiber neuropathy; the autonomic compromise is variable, and it may depend on the underlying disorder.

In small fiber neuropathy, distal sudomotor dysfunction is relevant, and it is useful for diagnosis, in combination with skin biopsy.

Management of small fiber neuropathy depends on adequate pain control and the recognition of a potential treatable cause.

Bibliography

1. Singer W, Spies J, McArthur J, Low J, Griffin J, Nickander K, et al. Prospective evaluation of somatic and autonomic small fibers in selected autonomic neuropathies. Neurology. 2004;62:612–8.
2. Devigili G, Tugnoli V, Penza P, Camozzi F, Lombardi R, Melli G, et al. The diagnostic criteria for small fibre neuropathy: from symptoms to neuropathology. Brain. 2008;13:1912–25.
3. Gibbons CH. Small fiber neuropathies. Continuum (Minneap Minn). 2014;20(5 Peripheral Nervous System Disorders):1398–412.
4. Themistocleous AC, Ramirez JD, Serra J, Bennett DL. The clinical approach to small fibre neuropathy and painful channelopathy. Pract Neurol. 2014;14:368–79.
5. Chan AC, Wilder-Smith EP. Small fiber neuropathy: Getting bigger! Muscle Nerve. 2016;53:671–82.

Chapter 12
Orthostatic Intolerance

Juan Idiaquez, Eduardo Benarroch, and Martin Nogues

Abstract Clinical case. Differential diagnosis: neurally mediated syncope (VVS, situational syncope), cardiac conditions, seizure disorder, metabolic, orthostatic hypotension, psychogenic pseudo syncope. Diagnosis: careful history taking, tilt table testing. Main manifestations of VVS: precipitant factors, prodromal features, characteristics of loss of consciousness period, post syncopal manifestations. Aggravating factors, associated conditions. Therapy: proper education of the patient, drug therapy. Prognosis: natural history of VVS.

‒‒‒‒‒‒‒‒
J. Idiaquez (✉)
Universidad de Valparaiso, Viña del Mar, Chile
e-mail: idiaquez@123.cl
E. Benarroch
Mayo Clinic, Rochester, MN, USA
e-mail: benarroch@mayo.edu
M. Nogues
Clinica Fleni, Buenos Aires, Argentina
e-mail: mnogues@fleni.org.ar

© Springer International Publishing AG 2018   109
J. Idiaquez et al. (eds.), *Evaluation and Management of Autonomic Disorders*,
https://doi.org/10.1007/978-3-319-72251-1_12

12.1   Case 1. Vasovagal Syncope

A 16-year-old woman, since the age of 13, began with dizziness and blurred vision on standing up, and she learned not to get up quickly. At that time she had a first episode of transient loss of consciousness while she was standing. She had prodromal symptoms including dizziness, sweating, fatigue, and odd sensation in the abdomen. Since that time she had suffered several similar episodes. During a venipuncture procedure (in supine position), the nurse observed that the patient fainted and showed brief multifocal jerks and urinary incontinence. There were no other specific situations that provoked syncope, and she did not have a family history of syncope. Medical evaluation showed normal EEG, ECG, ambulatory 24-h HR monitoring, and echocardiogram. Neurological evaluation: normal cognitive status. Cranial nerves: normal function. Motor examination: normal muscle strength and reflexes in upper and lower limbs. Sensory test: pinprick, temperature, and vibration on feet were normal. Tilt test did not show either orthostatic hypotension or postural tachycardia. After 25 min of tilting upward, the patient showed pre-syncope symptoms with hypotension. She recovered quickly on supine position.

12.2   Questions for Consideration

1. **Which conditions are suggested for the differential diagnosis on clinical evaluation?**
   Neurally mediated syncope: Vasovagal syncope (VVS) is the most frequent benign cause of transient loss of consciousness. Patients describe trigger factors (mainly prolonged standing or emotional distress) and prodromal symptoms. Situational syncope: while coughing, during defecation or micturition, during swallowing, and after meals. Carotid sinus hypersensitivity occurs mainly in elderly subjects.

Cardiac conditions: Arrhythmias like paroxysmal supraventricular and ventricular tachycardia, sinus node dysfunction, atrioventricular conduction disorder, and inherited conditions (Brugada and other syndromes). Severe structural heart disease can cause syncope: myocardial infarction, acute aortic dissection, obstructive cardiomyopathy, and others.

Seizure disorder: During an epileptic seizure, there is a generalized sudden tonic phase, followed by rhythmic clonic seizure, with cyanosis, tongue biting, and urinary incontinence. Postictal confusion is found.

Metabolic: During episodes of hypoglycemia, hypoxia, and hyperventilation with hypercapnia, patients may lose consciousness.

Orthostatic hypotension: Syncope may occur in non-neurogenic conditions like volume depletion, drugs causing hypovolemia, and others. Also syncope may occur in neurological disorders affecting central or peripheral sympathetic vasoconstrictor pathways.

Psychogenic pseudo-syncope: Patients report atypical prodromal symptoms like anxiety and abnormal breathing; the duration of the episode may be prolonged. Similarly a prolonged recovery period can occur. Patients with pseudo-syncope show many repeated faints in a short period of time. Occurrence of pseudo-syncope is more frequent in patients with history of VVS.

2. **Which investigations are useful in distinguishing among possible diagnoses?**
   Blood tests: complete cell count, thyroid function, creatinine, liver function, vitamin B12, and folate levels.
3. **What was the most likely diagnosis?**
   Neurally mediated vasovagal syncope.
4. **How was the patient treated?**
   The patient was treated with nonpharmacological measurement: education, avoidance of trigger factors, and diet with salt and adequate liquid ingestion.

12.3   Discussion

Our patient had a history of orthostatic intolerance for about 2 years, syncope triggered by two factors (postural and venipuncture), and prodromal symptoms compatible with VVS. Hypotensive response during tilt testing indicates that this patient had hypotensive/vasodepressor susceptibility. It is important to point out that hypotensive susceptibility showed by tilt testing can also be found in patients with cardiac syncope, so the test had a reduced specificity for diagnosis of VVS. Our patient showed generalized brief arrhythmic clonic jerking, with urinary incontinence, and a rapid recovery. This event raised the possibility of an epileptic seizure. The information given by a witness helps to differentiate between arrhythmic jerks occurring during syncope and rhythmic tonic clonic epileptic convulsion. Tongue biting, cyanosis, and postictal confusion are observed during epileptic seizures. Urinary incontinence during VVS occurs in about 25% of patients, and thus it is not useful to differentiate VVS from epilepsy. EEG during VVS shows a slow or a slow-flat-slow pattern due to a transient reduction of cerebral blood flow, while in an epileptic seizure, the EEG recording shows typical paroxysmal activity.

12.4   Relevant Aspect of Vasovagal Syncope

Etiology: The pathophysiological mechanisms of VVS are still not complete known. During the episode, all patients showed a transient loss of vasoconstrictor tone with BP fall (vasodepressor). In many patients, a transient increase of parasympathetic activity also occurs ranging from a mild bradycardia to an asystole (cardioinhibitory). The main afferent mechanisms of VVS are postural and emotional. In the postural type, the baroreflex mechanisms that increase systemic vascular resistance fail to maintain BP on standing. Also a reduction of cardiac output due to excessive splanchnic blood pooling can occur. In the emotional type, the afferent triggers are central pathways (cerebral cortex).

12.5   VVS Manifestations That Can Be Obtained by Careful History Taking

Precipitant factors: Syncope may be triggered by prolonged standing, emotional distress, fear, severe pain, venipuncture (seeing blood), warm or crowded environment, insufficient food intake, alcohol consumption, physical exercise (during or after), and others. It is important to consider that the characteristic of each trigger factor is wide-ranging, for instance, the duration of prolonged standing necessary to provoke syncope is different in each individual. In about half of the patients, more than one trigger factor is reported.

Prodromal features: Symptoms and signs due to autonomic activation and to retinal and cerebral hypoperfusion arise immediately, about 30–60 s before the patient faints. Main prodromal manifestations are lightheadedness (dizziness), blurred vision, facial pallor, sweating, fatigue, nausea, abdominal pain, palpitations, strong urge to defecate, sensation that environmental sounds are distant, buzzing in the ear, and feelings of cold or warm. If the patient reacts to these warning symptoms by sitting or lying down, the syncope can be avoided. These prodromal manifestations are present in younger patients, whereas older subjects reported prodromal symptoms less frequently.

Loss of consciousness period: This period takes only several seconds, but occasionally it can persist a longer time, especially if the patient remains on the standing position. Syncope occurs due to a transient and self-limited cerebral hypoperfusion. Some patients may present only a pre-syncope, with prodromal symptoms and signs together with an imminent sensation of syncope, but without loss of consciousness. Most of the patients are flaccid during syncope, and presences of arrhythmic myoclonic jerks are less frequent.

Post-syncopal manifestations: Recovery depends on the duration of low BP, mainly if the patient is quickly returned to the standing position and low BP does not recover. Among post-syncopal symptoms are weakness, fatigue than can last for hours or even days, persistence of facial pallor, nausea, yawning, and sweating.

Frequency of episodes: Isolated or few VVS faints can occur in healthy young subjects (between 10 and 20 years old), and it is not indicative of a neurological disease. In some subjects, a group of VVS occur in a short period of time (days or weeks), and then no new syncopes occur during the following years. Elderly subjects with a history of VVS at a young age can have it again. Recurrent VVS indicates the occurrence of three or more syncopes during the preceding 2 years. Repetition of VVS is associated with the number of attacks during childhood and adolescence.

Associated conditions: Syncope can occur during a migraine attack. In women with migraine, more VVS occurred compared with those without migraine. A family history of syncope may be obtained in some patients.

Uncommon presentation of VVS: Syncope in supine position during sleep time is rare, but it can occur in patients with a history of VVS during the day, triggered mainly by emotional distress. Possibly a central non-baroreflex dysfunction is associated with this condition. VVS may occur as a sudden fall without prodromal symptoms. If the patient suffers a retrograde amnesia, he/she cannot remember prodromal symptoms.

Diagnosis: A detailed history taking is the main tool for clinical diagnosis of VVS. Tilt table testing may reproduce symptoms and signs of VVS in about 40–50% of patients. When a drug (isoproterenol or nitroglycerine) is added to induce syncope, the test increases in sensitivity, but specificity is decreased. Tilt table testing is useful for detection of orthostatic hypotension and postural tachycardia and can also help to distinguish between VVS and other episodes, like epileptic attacks and pseudo-syncope.

Treatment and prognosis: Education must include (1) recognition of fainting trigger factors and ways to avoid them and (2) diet with increased adequate salt and fluid intake. Isometric exercise increases systemic BP, so if the patient performs isometric arm contractions during the beginning of prodromal symptoms, it can prevent the syncope. In most cases of vasovagal syncope, drug treatment is not necessary.

Fludrocortisone, midodrine, and serotonin reuptake inhibitors can be useful in patients with recurrent syncope. Cardiac pacemaker treatment for VVS is uncertain, and the possible benefit of pacing for patients with cardioinhibitory type of VVS and asystole is debatable.

12.6 Key Points

In VVS, there occurs a transient loss of consciousness due to cerebral hypoperfusion. Immediately before syncope, there are symptoms due to autonomic activation and to cerebral and retinal hypoperfusion.

VVS is the most frequent cause of syncope in young subjects, while in elderly subjects, cardiac disorders and orthostatic hypotension are common causes.

A careful and detailed history is the main diagnostic tool for VVS, comprising recognition of precipitating factors, prodromal symptoms, characteristics of the episode, and recovery period.

Initial evaluation of VVS includes an ECG and study of blood pressure and heart rate change on standing. Tilt table testing may help to reproduce the syncope, but its sensitivity and specificity are limited.

Therapeutic management for VVS must consider a proper education of the patient. Medication may be useful in some patients with recurrent syncope.

Abstract Clinical case. Differential diagnosis of conditions presenting with postural tachycardia: POTS, physical deconditioning, anxiety and panic attacks, systemic disorders, inappropriate sinus tachycardia syndrome. Diagnosis: history taking, ECG, plasma noradrenaline, tilt table testing. Main manifestations of POTS: orthostatic and non orthostatic symptoms. Pathophysiological characteristics of neurogenic and hyperadrenergic types. Therapy: proper education of the patient, drug therapy. Prognosis.

12.7   Case 2. Postural Orthostatic Tachycardia Syndrome (POTS)

A 22-year-old woman, over the past 10 months, has experienced symptoms while she was standing. The patient referred lightheadedness, fatigue, and palpitations. No history of a recent viral disease was reported. These symptoms became worse, and she noticed intolerance to mild physical exercise and to warm environments. She presented several episodes of pre-syncope. She complained of abdominal pain with diarrhea, trouble in falling sleep, difficulty concentrating, and irritability. She suffers an acute episode of chest pain and palpitations. A medical evaluation showed normal physical examination including motor and sensory evaluation, supine BP 110/60 mmHg, and supine HR 72 beats/min. ECG, 24 ECG Holter monitoring, and echocardiogram were all normal. Blood test: fasting glucose, complete cell count, thyroid function, creatinine, and electrolytes—all were normal. She was diagnosed with an anxiety disorder, and she was sent to psychotherapy. Her orthostatic intolerance symptoms and fatigue continued; she felt better on supine position. A tilt table testing showed postural tachycardia (orthostatic change = 42 bpm), without BP change. Plasma noradrenaline on supine = 210 pg/mL and standing = 445 pg/mL (normal). Cardiovascular autonomic testing: Valsalva normal phases II and IV. Cardiovagal test (deep breathing): normal HR change. Sudomotor: Quantitative sudomotor axon reflex test (QSART) showed normal sweating in the ankle.

12.8   Questions for Consideration

1. **Which conditions for the differential diagnosis are suggested by clinical evaluation?**
   POTS: There are chronic symptoms (>6 months) of orthostatic intolerance, associated with postural tachycardia, without orthostatic hypotension. Other symptoms like fatigue, gastrointestinal, urinary, migraine, sleep disorders,

and anxiety are present. Main pathophysiological mechanisms described in POTS are neuropathic (distal sympathetic denervation) and hyperadrenergic types.

Conditions Other than POTS, Which May Present with Chronic Orthostatic Tachycardia

Physical deconditioning: It may occur in the context of a short or prolonged period of inactivity or bed rest, and it is more frequent in elderly subjects. Also, it may be induced by space flight. Cardiovascular deconditioning includes a reduction of spontaneous baroreflex sensitivity, supine, and postural tachycardia. Patients show orthostatic symptoms.

Anxiety and panic attacks: Patients with generalized anxiety or panic crisis may show faster HR during the day. During tilt table testing, patients may present anxiety symptoms associated with a transient postural tachycardia (usually for <10 min).

Systemic disorders: Thyrotoxicosis—there is a cardiac sympathetic activation, and also thyroid hormone may have direct action on sinoatrial node, causing tachycardia. Pheochromocytoma: patients present with crisis of hypertension and tachycardia symptoms, while standing or in lying position. High supine plasma and urine norepinephrine levels are found.

Inappropriate sinus tachycardia syndrome: Supine sinus HR is elevated >100 bpm and mean 24 h HR >90 bpm. A cardiac structural or a systemic disorder is absent. Symptoms may be similar to POTS and are triggered by both emotional and physiological stresses, while in POTS, symptoms are induced by orthostatic stress and relief on supine position.

2. **Which investigations were useful to distinguish among possible diagnosis?**
   Blood test: fasting glucose, complete cell count, thyroid function, creatinine, electrolytes and supine, and standing plasma noradrenaline—all were normal. ECG, 24 ECG Holter monitoring, and echocardiogram were all normal. Tilt table testing showed orthostatic tachycardia.

3. **What was the most likely diagnosis?**
   POTS.
4. **How was the patient treated?**
   Education, psychotherapy, sufficient hydration and salt intake, avoidance of triggering factors, and low dose of propranolol.

12.9   Discussion

Our patient had a history of chronic orthostatic and non-orthostatic symptoms, the tilt table testing showed orthostatic tachycardia without BP fall. The patient referred several episodes of pre-syncope; about 30% of patients with POTS also present typical VVS. She showed anxiety symptoms; it is known that POTS patients may present anxiety and panic disorders. The present case did not show excessive increase of plasma noradrenaline on standing; possibly this case is not related with any hyperadrenergic condition. Our patient did not present a painful small fiber neuropathy, and both cardiovagal and distal sudomotor function were preserved. In POTS, about 50% of the patients may show abnormal sudomotor tests in the legs. It is relevant that sudomotor dysfunction in POTS may also present a patchy or a proximal distribution. Cardiovagal denervation occurs only in about 10% of patients. It is difficult to classify a patient according to a specific pathophysiological type of POTS. Neuropathic and hyperadrenergic mechanisms can coexist in the same individual.

12.10   Relevant Aspect of POTS

Pathophysiology: POTS is a chronic and heterogeneous syndrome; abnormal HR rise on standing may result from varied pathophysiological mechanisms: (1) Neuropathic POTS (restricted autonomic neuropathy): there is moderate impairment of distal sympathetic vasoconstriction on standing, leading to venous pooling in lower limbs and splanchnic vessels. It may be caused by a small fiber neuropathy. There are both experimental and clinical studies that suggest distal sympathetic denervation: hypersensitivity to infusion of norepinephrine into veins of the foot, reduced norepinephrine spillover during sympathetic activation, abnormal cardiac sympathetic imaging, and abnormal distal sudomotor tests. (2) Hyperadrenergic type: there is an excessive sympathetic response on standing, and upright plasma noradrenaline is elevated ($\geq$600 pg/mL). This type may be primary; it is important to consider secondary causes of sympathetic hyperactivity like effect of drug treatment, hypovolemia, thyrotoxicosis, pheochromocytoma, mast cell activation, and familial norepinephrine transport deficiency. Many patients with POTS show blood volume reduction, due to an abnormal activation of the renin-angiotensin system. This hypovolemia aggravates symptoms of orthostatic intolerance. Also, autoimmune POTS with elevated autoantibodies to ganglionic ACh receptors and α1-adrenergic receptors have been reported.

12.11   POTS Manifestations

Clinical: More than 75% of patients are female; it occurs in most patients between the ages of 15 and 25 years. Half of the patients report a previous viral disease. Some patients have a family history of POTS.   Clinical presentation of POTS includes varied chronic symptoms: (1) orthostatic intolerance, symptoms include both due to cerebral hypoperfusion and sympathetic activation (lightheadedness (dizziness), blurred vision, mental clouding, palpitation, chest pain, dyspnea, and tremulousness, among others). (2) Non-orthostatic symptoms: fatigue, bloating, nausea, abdominal pain and diarrhea, bladder symptoms, migraine, and sleep disorder. Symptoms can worsen by prolonged standing, hot environment, menses, after a heavy meal, alcohol intake, and exercise. Physical signs: patients may show neurological signs of small fiber neuropathy, and also skin changes (acrocyanosis) and edema in lower limbs can be found. Also cold and wet hands are caused by sympathetic overactivity.

Associated conditions: Patients with POTS may display several associated conditions like chronic fatigue syndrome, joint hypermobility (Ehlers-Danlos syndrome), anxiety, depression, sleep disturbances, migraine, and type I Chiari malformation associated with syringomyelia.

Diagnosis: History taking—orthostatic intolerance symptoms must have lasted for more than 6 months. Symptoms occurring while the patient is in upright position must improve when he is lying down. HR increases ≥ 30 bpm within 10 min of standing and more than 40 bpm in youngers (12–19 years old), from a supine position (during tilt table testing or active standing). HR usually may increase ≥ 120 beats/min (bpm) on standing. There is not postural blood pressure change. Blood test: fasting glucose, complete cell count, thyroid function, creatinine, electrolytes, and supine and standing plasma noradrenaline. Additional blood testing depends on specific suspected condition. Cardiac disorders, systemic condition (anemia, dehydration, hyperthyroidism, and hyperadrenergic conditions), or any drug treatment that predispose to postural tachycardia (diuretics, vasodilators, sympathomimetic) must be excluded.

12.12   Treatment and Prognosis

Management of POTS patients is a challenge, due to the multifactorial causes of the symptomatology.

1. Nonpharmacological measures: A comprehensive education about the characteristic of symptoms is useful for managing patient expectation. Adequate hydration and salt intake support garments, avoidance of aggravating factors, and short-term grading exercise program. Non-upright exercises (swimming, recumbent cycles) are useful.
2. Pharmacological treatment: Drug therapy for POTS depends on the different factors like hypovolemia, impaired peripheral vasoconstriction, increased venous

pooling, and hyperadrenergic condition, which contribute to symptoms. In patients with hypovolemia, fludrocortisone, midodrine, and pyridostigmine may be useful for orthostatic symptoms. A low dose of propranolol (patient may have a β-adrenoceptor supersensitivity) is useful to alleviate symptoms caused by standing tachycardia. Side effects of each drug must be considered. Drug therapy for one symptom may have a negative influence on other clinical manifestation: fludrocortisone on headache, midodrine on gastrointestinal and urinary symptoms, pyridostigmine on chronic diarrhea, and propranolol on chronic fatigue, among others. No specific drug is consistently effective.

12.13   Key Points

POTS is a multifactorial clinical syndrome that mostly affects young and middle-aged women.

Main pathophysiological mechanisms that contribute to POTS are neuropathic type (distal sympathetic denervation) and hyperadrenergic type.

POTS presents with multiple symptoms including orthostatic and non-orthostatic manifestations; this mixed symptomatology is relevant for diagnosis and treatment.

Differential diagnosis of POTS must consider cardiac disorders and systemic causes of excessive sympathetic activation.

Management of POTS: Nonpharmacological is central for controlling patient expectation; pharmacological therapy must be focused on each patient symptomatology.

Bibliography

1. Sheldon RS, Grubb BP, Olshansky B, Shen WK, Calkins H, Brignole M, et al. 2015 heart rhythm society expert consensus statement on the diagnosis and treatment of postural tachycardia syndrome, inappropriate sinus tachycardia, and vasovagal syncope. Heart Rhythm. 2015;12:e41–63.

2. Wieling W, Thijs RD, van Dijk N, Wilde AA, Benditt DG, van Dijk JG. Symptoms and signs of syncope: a review of the link between physiology and clinical clues. Brain. 2009;132:2630–42.
3. Wieling W, van Dijk N, de Lange FJ, Olde Nordkamp LR, Thijs RD, van Dijk JG, Linzer M, Sutton R. History taking as a diagnostic test in patients with syncope: developing expertise in syncope. Eur Heart J. 2015;36:277–80.
4. Sutton R, Brignole M. Twenty-eight years of research permits reinterpretation of tilt-testing: hypotensive susceptibility rather than diagnosis. Eur Heart J. 2014;35:2211–2.
5. Thieben MJ, Sandroni P, Sletten DM, Benrud-Larson LM, Fealey RD, et al. Postural orthostatic tachycardia syndrome: the Mayo clinic experience. Mayo Clin Proc. 2007;82:308–13.
6. Benarroch EE. Postural tachycardia syndrome: a heterogeneous and multifactorial disorder. Mayo Clin Proc. 2012;87:1214–25.
7. Jones PK, Shaw BH, Raj SR. Clinical challenges in the diagnosis and management of postural tachycardia syndrome. Pract Neurol. 2016;16:431–8.

Chapter 13
Autonomic Hyperactivity

Juan Idiaquez, Eduardo Benarroch, and Martin Nogues

13.1 Case 1. Paroxysmal Sympathetic Hyperactivity in Severe Brain Injury

A 20-year-old man was involved in a car crash. He lost consciousness and he was transferred to the hospital. He underwent nasotracheal intubation. Physical examination showed a comatose patient (Glasgow scale = 5). To painful stimuli, he did not open his eyes but showed a reflex motor response with extensor posturing. His pupils were isochoric, without fotomotor response. A computed tomography (CT) of the head showed several bilateral intracerebral hemorrhages.

J. Idiaquez (✉)
Universidad de Valparaiso, Viña del Mar, Chile
e-mail: idiaquez@123.cl

E. Benarroch
Mayo Clinic, Rochester, MN, USA
e-mail: benarroch@mayo.edu

M. Nogues
Clinica Fleni, Buenos Aires, Argentina
e-mail: mnogues@fleni.org.ar

© Springer International Publishing AG 2018   123
J. Idiaquez et al. (eds.), *Evaluation and Management of Autonomic Disorders*,
https://doi.org/10.1007/978-3-319-72251-1_13

Cervical X showed no fracture. All body CT scanning was normal. He was admitted to intensive unit care for mechanical ventilation. Intracranial pressure monitoring was installed (ICP). During the following two days, the patient remained in coma, and the ICP rose up to 22 mmHg. He was treated with Mannitol and hyperventilation. Three days later, he presented several episodes of bilateral extension posture with profuse sweating and hyperthermia. Cardiovascular monitoring showed BP and HR elevation during the episodes. Some paroxysms occurred spontaneously, but others were provoked by a sound and tactile stimulation. An electroencephalogram during the episode showed no epileptic discharges. Blood and urine cultures were negative. Cerebrospinal fluid (CSF) was normal. Chest X-ray was normal.

13.2   Questions for Consideration

1. **What conditions can present with paroxysmal autonomic hyperactivity?**
   Paroxysmal sympathetic hyperactivity (PSH) due to severe acute brain injuries: Patients show repeated paroxysms of hypertension, tachycardia, hyperthermia, excessive sweating, tachypnea, and descerebrate posturing. Causes of PSH are traumatic brain injury (TBI), hypoxia, subarachnoid hemorrhage, brainstem stroke, acute hydrocephalus, tumors, hypoglycemia, and infections.
   Autonomic hyperactivity associated with subacute encephalopathy: (1) Autoimmune disorders: limbic encephalitis (VGKC, LGI1) manifestations are confusion, working memory loss, psychiatric disturbances, seizures, and sympathetic hyperactivity. Morvan syndrome (VGKC-Caspr2) manifestations are severe insomnia, hallucinations, neuromyotonia, myoclonus, and sympathetic hyperactivity. Anti-NMDA receptor encephalitis is characterized by cognitive dysfunction, abnormal behavior, seizures, movement disorders, central hypoventilation, and sympathetic and parasympathetic hyperactivity. Stiff man syndrome (GAD or

GyR1R): there is a diminished inhibitory action of GABA on motor and autonomic pathways in the brain stem and spinal cord. Patients show episodes of muscle rigidity, hypertension, tachycardia, hyperhidrosis, and pupillary dilatation. (2) Delirium tremens due to alcohol withdrawn: patients present symptoms of anxiety, hallucinations, hypertension, tachycardia, and hyperhidrosis. (3) Fatal insomnia (autosomal prion disorder and occasionally sporadic): patients present progressive sleep disturbances, hypertension, sweating, excessive salivation, and lacrimation. Later stages show motor symptoms (pyramidal signs, myoclonus, dysmetria, and abnormal gait).

Autonomic dysreflexia in spinal cord injury: Due to cervical or high thoracic spinal cord (above T5) injury. Immediately after the injury, there is a transient period of motor and autonomic hypoexitability (acute spinal shock), lasting from days to weeks. After that, autonomic dysreflexia may occur; it comprises of a massive sympathetic reflex discharge, provoked by stimuli (below the level of the lesion). There is a severe hypertension that can lead to hemorrhagic stroke, myocardial infarction, pulmonary edema, and renal insufficiency.

Peripheral nervous system disorders: Baroreflex failure— due to a lesion of the afferent limb of the baroreflex at the level of carotid sinus, afferent pathways, or medulla. Patients present episodes of severe hypertension, tachycardia, excessive sweating, palpitations, headache, and flushing. A minority of patients show episodes of hypotension or bradycardia. Patients with baroreflex failure show absence of bradycardia in response to BP rise and absence of tachycardia in response to BP fall. In familial dysautonomia (hereditary sensory and autonomic neuropathy HSAN type III), patient shows orthostatic hypotension and paroxysms of hypertension due to a congenital dysfunction of the afferent limb of the baroreflex. Patient phenotypes include decreased pain and thermal sensation, abnormal swallowing, diminished taste sensation, smooth tongue due to absent fungiform papillae, and absence of tears. In Guillain-Barre syndrome and porphyria, episodes of hypertension may occur.

Other conditions: Pheochromocytoma and episodic hypothermia (agenesis of corpus callosum). Focal cortical disorders: insular stroke and temporal lobe seizures. Iatrogenic disorders: neuroleptic malignant syndrome, serotonin syndrome, anticholinergic syndrome, and malignant hyperthermia. Drug intoxication: cocaine and amphetamine. Drug withdrawal: alcohol, baclofen, and opioid. Biological toxin: tetanus and Irukandji syndrome caused by jellyfish sting.

2. **Which investigations were useful to distinguish among possible diagnosis?**
   Medical history, physical examination, and CT scan showed a severe TBI. Paroxysms of hypertension, tachycardia, fever, hyperhidrosis, tachypnea, and decerebrate posturing. EEG did not show epileptic discharges. Tests did not show any infectious disease.
3. **What was the most likely diagnosis?**
   PSH due to severe TBI.
4. **How was the patient treated?**
   He received labetalol and morphine.

13.3   Discussion

Our patient showed repeated paroxysms of excessive sympathetic activation and extensor posturing during the early phase of a severe TBI; epileptic seizures, infective disorder, and drug withdrawal were excluded. These features supported the diagnosis of PSH; in this condition, symptoms of sympathetic overactivity are predominant. Sympathetic paroxysms are the main manifestation in conditions such as encephalopathies, peripheral nerve disorders, and autonomic dysreflexia. Symptoms of mixed sympathetic and parasympathetic activation are less frequent. Symptoms of parasympathetic hyperactivity such as bradyarrhythmia, diarrhea, lacrimation, and excessive salivation can occur in Guillain-Barre, in some autoimmune encephalitis, and in familial fatal insomnia among others.

13.4   Relevant Aspect of PSH

Clinical Manifestations

PSH occurs in young patients; the main cause in adults is a severe TBI, and less common are severe hypoxia and stroke. In children, PSH is more common in hypoxia and encephalitis. Paroxysms of hypertension, tachycardia, tachypnea, hyperthermia, hyperhidrosis, and extensor posturing may be triggered by noxious and non-noxious external stimuli. Episodes occur mainly during the first week following the TBI, but also a minority can occur in a late phase during rehabilitation. Episodes can occur one to three times per day, and the duration of each paroxysm is from a short period to 10 h. The total duration of the paroxysmal period is variable, from less than 2 weeks to several months. The exact pathophysiology is debatable, possibly a disconnection of forebrain (insula, cingulate cortex) inhibitory influences with the hypothalamus and upper brainstem sympathoexcitatory pathways. Excessive sympathetic overactivity can lead to intracranial hemorrhage, brain edema, congestive heart failure, Takotsubo syndrome, and neurogenic pulmonary edema.

Diagnosis

Medical history and physical examination are relevant. The diagnosis of PSH in patients with TBI requires the presence of the following features: episodes of sympathetic overactivity to normally non-noxious stimuli; features persist for more than 3 consecutive days and follow for more than 2 weeks. Sympathetic paroxysms occur in absence of other presumed causes.

Treatment and Prognosis

Therapy of patients with sympathetic hyperactivity is focused on (1) management of sympathetic activation, (2) reduction of the end-organ response to sympathetic activation, and

(3) suppression of sensory afferent that triggered sympathetic paroxysm. Most patients require a multiple drug treatment. Propranolol, labetalol, metoprolol, and clonidine are useful to treat hypertension and tachycardia. Morphine and fentanyl may suppress the sympathetic responses triggered by external stimuli. Bromocriptine, gabapentin, and baclofen are neuromodulators that help to control the sympathetic storm. PSH is an independent risk factor for worse outcome in patients who have had a brain injury.

13.5   Key Points

Autonomic (mainly sympathetic) hyperactivity is a potential life-threatening condition that can affect different organs.

Paroxysms of sympathetic hyperactivity are manifested by hypertension, tachycardia, arrhythmias, excessive sweating, and abnormal regulation of temperature; symptoms may be triggered by noxious and non-noxious external stimuli.

Autonomic hyperactivity may occur in acute or subacute neurological disorders; common causes are severe brain trauma, subarachnoid hemorrhage, autonomic dysreflexia in spinal cord injury, Guillain-Barre, and iatrogenic disorders.

Autonomic hyperactivity may be a prominent manifestation of autoimmune and prion disorders.

Sepsis, drug intoxication, or withdrawal should always be excluded in patients with autonomic hyperactivity.

Management in an intensive unit care, multiple drug treatment focused in the different pathophysiological mechanisms, early recognition, and elimination of triggering stimuli are relevant.

Bibliography

1. Ketch T, Biaggioni I, Robertson R, Robertson D. Four faces of baroreflex failure: hypertensive crisis, volatile hypertension, orthostatic tachycardia, and malignant vagotonia. Circulation. 2002;105:2518–23.

2. Perkes I, Baguley IJ, Nott MT, Menon DK. A review of paroxysmal sympathetic hyperactivity after acquired brain injury. Ann neurol. 2010;68:126–35.
3. Meyfroidt G, Baguley IJ, Menon DK. Paroxysmal sympathetic hyperactivity: the storm after acute brain injury. Lancet Neurol. 2017;16:721–9.
4. Graus F, Titulaer MJ, Balu R, Benseler S, Bien CG, Cellucci T, et al. A clinical approach to diagnosis of autoimmune encephalitis. Lancet Neurol. 2016;15:391–404.
5. Eldahan KC, Rabchevsky AG. Autonomic dysreflexia after spinal cord injury: systemic pathophysiology and methods of management. Auton Neurosci. 2017.
6. Norcliffe-Kaufmann L, Kaufmann H. Familial dysautonomia (Riley-Day syndrome): when baroreceptor feedback fails. Auton Neurosci. 2012;172:26–30.

Index

© Springer International Publishing AG 2018   131
J. Idiaquez et al. (eds.), *Evaluation and Management of Autonomic Disorders*,
https://doi.org/10.1007/978-3-319-72251-1